106

Anaesthesiology and Resuscitation
Anaesthesiologie und Wiederbelebung
Anesthésiologie et Réanimation

Editors:

R. Frey, Mainz · F. Kern, St. Gallen
O. Mayrhofer, Wien

Managing Editor: H. Bergmann, Linz

Etomidate

An Intravenous Hypnotic Agent

First Report on Clinical and Experimental Experience

Edited by A. Doenicke

With 59 Figures

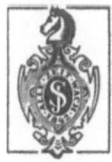

Springer-Verlag
Berlin Heidelberg GmbH 1977

ISBN 978-3-540-08485-3   ISBN 978-3-642-66787-9 (eBook)
DOI 10.1007/978-3-642-66787-9

2127/3140-543210

Preface

The question how to induce general anaesthesia without problems
has been asked repeatedly by anaesthetists and pharmacologists.

P.A. JANSSEN developed etomidate and published this substance in
1971 as "a potent short-acting and relatively atoxic intravenous
hypnotic agent in rats".

In 1974 after several years of experimental and clinical trial
the barbiturate-free hypnotic etomidate (soon marketed as
Hypnomidate) was introduced to numerous auditors at the occasion
of the IV. European Congress of Anaesthesiologists in Madrid.

As the authors extended their essays, the actuality of the present
book is given.

The conclusion mentions the new solution of etomidate base in
35 % propylene glycol.

It is expected that the disadvantageous effects - venous pain
during injection and associated involuntary muscle movements -
will largely be eliminated by using the new formula of etomidate
after premedication of fentanyl.

München, August 1977   Alfred DOENICKE

Table of Contents

The Experimental Pharmacology of Etomidate, a New Potent,
Short-Acting Intravenous Hypnotic
(R.S. RENEMAN and P.A. JANSSEN) 1

Protein Binding of Etomidate
(G.A. MANNES and A. DOENICKE) 6

The Effect of Intra-Arterial Injection of Etomidate and
Thiopental on the Skeletal Muscle- and Arterial Wall-Structures
(R.S. RENEMAN, F. VERHEYEN, R. KRUGER, W. VAN GERVEN and
M. BORGES) 9

Interaction between Etomidate and the Antihypertensive Agents
Propanolol and ∝-Methyl-Dopa
(R.S. RENEMAN, W. VAN GERVEN and R. KRUGER) 15

Teratogenicity of Etomidate
(A. DOENICKE and M. HAEHL) 23

Etomidate, A New Hypnotic Agent for Intravenous Application
(A. DOENICKE) 25

The EEG after Etomidate
(J. KUGLER, A. DOENICKE and M. LAUB) 31

A Comparison of the Acute Effects of Intravenous Induction
Agents (Thiopentone, Methohexitone, Propanidid, Althesin,
Ketamine, Piritramide and Etomidate) on Haemodynamics and
Myocardial Oxygen Consumption in Dogs
(D. PATSCHKE, J.B. BRÜCKNER, J.W. GETHMANN, J. TARNOW and
A. WEYMAR) 49

Haemodynamic Effects of Etomidate - a New Hypnotic - in Patients
with Myocardial Insufficiency
(G. HEMPELMANN, W. OSTER, S. PIEPENBROCK and G. KARLICZEK) .. 72

VIII

Haemodynamics, Myocardial Function, Oxygen Requirement, and
Oxygen Supply of the Human Heart after Administration of
Etomidate
(D. KETTLER, H. SONNTAG, U. WOLFRAM-DONATH, H.J. HOEFT,
D. REGENSBURGER and H.D. SCHENK) 81

Experimental Investigations on the Direct Effect of Etomidate
on Myocardial Contractility
(K.-J. FISCHER and H. MARQUORT) 95

The Influence of R 26 490 (Etomidate Sulfate) on Ventilation and
Gas Exchange
(B. MARQUARDT, H. WAIBEL and J.B. BRÜCKNER) 113

A Comparative Study of Blood Gases and Haemodynamics Using the
New Hypnotic Etomidate, CT 1341, Methohexitone, Propanidid and
Thiopentone
(W. HEMPELMANN, G. HEMPELMANN and S. PIEPENBROCK) 119

The Use of Etomidate as an Induction Agent in Fentanyl Analgesia
(Z. KALENDA) 130

Etomidate Anaesthesia for Cardioversion
(A. WEYMAR, D. PATSCHKE, J. TARNOW and J.B. BRÜCKNER) 140

Etomidate and Fentanyl for Emergency Anaesthesia in Acute Bleeding
with Haemorrhagic Shock
(M. ZINDLER) 144

Clinical Experience with Etomidate in Diagnostical Interventions
and Operations of Short Duration
(A. DOENICKE, W. SPIESS, B. GROTE and J. ARANOJI) 146

Etomidate as "A New Drug in Intravenous Anaesthesia" (Conclusion)
(A. DOENICKE) 152

Contributors

ARANOJI, J., Dr. med., Chirurgische Poliklinik der Universität,
  Anaesthesie-Abteilung, Pettenkofer Str. 8a, 8000 München 2

BORGES, M., Dr. med., Janssen Pharmaceutica n.v., B-2340 Beerse,
  Belgien

BRÜCKNER, J.B., Prof. Dr. med., Klinikum Westend der Freien
  Universität Berlin, Institut für Anaesthesiologie, Spandauer
  Damm 130, 1000 Berlin 19

DOENICKE, A., Prof. Dr. med., Chirurgische Poliklinik der Universität, Anaesthesie-Abteilung, Pettenkofer Str. 8a, 8000 München 2

FISCHER, K.-J., Dr. med., Medizinische Fakultät der Christian-
  Albrechts-Universität, Abteilung für Anaesthesiologie, Olshausen-
  str. 40-60, 2300 Kiel

GETHMANN, J.W., Dr. med., Klinikum Westend der Freien Universität
  Berlin, Institut für Anaesthesiologie, Spandauer Damm 130,
  1000 Berlin 19

GROTE, B., Dr. med., Chirurgische Poliklinik der Universität,
  Anaesthesie-Abteilung, Pettenkofer Str. 8a, 8000 München 2

HAEHL, M., Dr. med., Chirurgische Poliklinik der Universität,
  Anaesthesie-Abteilung, Pettenkofer Str. 8a, 8000 München 2

HEMPELMANN, G., Prof. Dr. med., Medizinische Hochschule Hannover,
  Institut für Anaesthesiologie, Karl-Wiechert-Allee 9,
  3000 Hannover 61

HEMPELMANN, W., Dr. med., Medizinische Hochschule Hannover,
  Institut für Anaesthesiologie, Karl-Wiechert-Allee 9,
  3000 Hannover 61

HOEFT, H.J., Medizinische Fakultät der Georg-August-Universität,
  Institut für klinische Anaesthesie, Goßler Str. 10, 3400 Göttingen

JANSSEN, P.A.J., Dr. med., Janssen Pharmaceutica n.v., B-2340
  Beerse, Belgien

KALENDA, Z., Dr. med., Academisch Ziekenhuis Utrecht, Instituut
  voor Anaesthesiologie van den Rijksuniversiteit, Catharijne-
  singel 101, Utrecht, Holland

KARLICZEK, G., Dr. med., Medizinische Hochschule Hannover,
  Institut für Anaesthesiologie, Karl-Wiechert-Allee 9,
  3000 Hannover 61

KETTLER, D., Prof. Dr. med., Medizinische Fakultät der Georg-
  August-Universität, Institut für klinische Anaesthesie,
  Goßler Str. 10, 3400 Göttingen

KRUGER, R., Dr. med., Department of Physiology, Biomedical Center,
  Medical Faculty Maastricht, Beeldsnijdersdreef 101, Maastricht,
  Niederlande

MANNES, G.A., Chirurgische Poliklinik der Universität, Anaesthesie-
  Abteilung, Pettenkofer Str. 8a, 8000 München 2

MARQUARDT, B., Chefarzt Dr. med., Johanna-Etienne-Krankenhaus,
  Am Hasenberg 46, 4040 Neuss

MARQUORT, H., Dr. med., Medizinische Fakultät der Christian-
  Albrechts-Universität, Abteilung für Anaesthesiologie, Olshau-
  senstr. 40-60, 2300 Kiel

OSTER, W., Dr. med., Medizinische Hochschule Hannover, Institut
  für Anaesthesiologie, Karl-Wiechert-Allee 9, 3000 Hannover 61

PATSCHKE, D., Prof. Dr. med., Anaesthesie-Abteilung, Klinikum der
  Justus-Liebig-Universität, Klinikstraße 29, 6300 Giessen

PIEPENBROCK, S., Dr. med., Medizinische Hochschule Hannover,
  Institut für Anaesthesiologie, Karl-Wiechert-Allee 9,
  3000 Hannover 61

REGENSBURGER, D., Dr. med., Priv. Doz., Medizinische Fakultät der
  Georg-August-Universität, Institut für klinische Anaesthesie,
  Goßler Str. 10, 3400 Göttingen

RENEMAN, R., Prof. Dr. med., Department of Physiology, Biomedical
  Center, Medical Faculty Maastricht, Beeldsnijdersdreef 101,
  Maastricht, Niederlande

SONNTAG, H., Prof. Dr. med., Medizinische Fakultät der Georg-
  August-Universität, Institut für klinische Anaesthesie, Goßler
  Str. 10, 3400 Göttingen

SPIESS, W., Chefarzt Dr. med., Anaesthesie-Abteilung, Kreiskranken-
  haus, Seilerweg 29, 6430 Bad Hersfeld

SCHENK, H.D., Dr. med., Medizinische Fakultät der Georg-August-
  Universität, Institut für klinische Anaesthesie, Goßler Str. 10,
  3400 Göttingen

TARNOW, J., Dr. med., Priv. Doz., Klinikum Westend der Freien
  Universität Berlin, Institut für Anaesthesiologie, Spandauer
  Damm 130, 1000 Berlin 19

VAN GERVEN, W., Dr. med., Janssen Pharmaceutica n.v., B-2340 Beerse, Belgien

VERHEYEN, F., Dr. med., Janssen Pharmaceutica n.v., B-2340 Beerse, Belgien

VAN ZWIETEN, P.A., Prof. Dr. med., Universität Amsterdam, Laboratorium voor Biofarmacie, Amsterdam, Niederlande

WAIBEL, H., Dr. med., Krankenhaus Spandau, Örtl. Bereich Havelhöhe, Lynarstr. 12, 1000 Berlin 20

WEYMAR, A., Dr. med., Klinikum Westend der Freien Universität Berlin, Institut für Anaesthesiologie, Spandauer Damm 130, 1000 Berlin 19

WOLFRAM-DONATH, U., Medizinische Fakultät der Georg-August-Universität, Institut für klinische Anaesthesie, Goßler Str. 10, 3400 Göttingen

ZINDLER, M., Prof. Dr. med., Institut für Anaesthesiologie der Universität Düsseldorf, Moorenstr. 5, 4000 Düsseldorf

The Experimental Pharmacology of Etomidate, a New Potent, Short-Acting Intravenous Hypnotic

R.S. Reneman and P.A.J. Janssen

Chemistry

Etomidate (R-(+)-ethyl-1-(1-phenylethyl)-1H-imidazole-5-carb-oxylate), which was developed in our laboratories, is a new, potent, short-acting and safe intravenous hypnotic, with the following structural formula:

Etomidate is supplied as the sulfate (molecular weight; 342.36) and is dissolved in 1.8 mg $Na_2 HPO_4 \cdot 12 H_2O$ and 2.2 mg $Na H_2 PO_4 \cdot 1 H_2O$ with 4.2 % glucose in a concentration of 1.5 mg etomidate base per ml (pH about 3.4).

General Pharmacology

On rapid (2 sec) intravenous injection in rats, etomidate (ED_{50} = 0.57 mg/kg) is approx. 6 times more potent than methohexital (ED_{50} = 3.51 mg/kg) and about 25 times more potent than propanidid and thiopental (ED_{50}'s = 13.4 mg/kg). The safety margin (LD_{50}/ED_{50}) in rats is for etomidate 26.0, for methohexital 9.5, for propanidid 6.7 and for thiopental 4.6. The potency and toxicity of etomidate increase slightly with increasing injection rates without affecting the safety margin significantly (JANSSEN et al., 1971, 1975).

Etomidate is a pure hypnotic and has no analgesic activity. It has a rapid onset of action and induces hypnosis within one minute. In rats, guinea pigs and dogs, the duration of hypnosis with etomidate is dose-dependent, the duration of the hypnotic effect being doubled when the dose is doubled. With lower body weights

higher doses in mg/kg are required for inducing hypnosis of
comparable duration. No tolerance is observed after repeated
administration. The time needed to recover from hypnosis is short
and related to the duration of the hypnosis. The recovery-time is
approx. 4 to 5 times the duration of the hypnotic effect at low
doses and about 1.5 times the duration of the hypnotic effect at
high doses (JANSSEN et al., 1971, 1975).

Toxicology and Teratology

ECG, haematological and biochemical analyses, urinanalysis and
histopathology fail to reveal any drug-related adverse effects
after the daily intravenous injection of etomidate for 3 weeks
in rats (highest dose 5.0 mg/kg) and 2 weeks in dogs (highest
dose 1.5 mg/kg).

Etomidate is devoid of any teratogenic effect in rats and in white
rabbits of the New-Zealand strain. The highest dose of etomidate
given to rats was 5.0 mg/kg i.v. daily from day 6 through day 15
of pregnancy and to rabbits 4.5 mg/kg i.v. daily from day 6
through day 18 of pregnancy (JANSSEN et al., 1975).

Distribution and Metabolism

During the first 30 min after administration in humans, the
plasma level of unchanged etomidate decreases rapidly and then
more slowly with a half-life time of 75 min (HEYKANTS et al.,
1973). During transport etomidate is bound to the plasma-proteins
(MEULDERMANS and HEYKANTS, 1976). Directly after intravenous
injection in rats the plasma levels of etomidate drop quickly
and the hypnotic penetrates the brain rapidly since the levels
are maximal within one min after administration. This finding
corresponds to the fast onset of the hypnotic effect as observed
in animals and humans. In rats, the minimum level of etomidate
sufficient to induce hypnosis can be estimated at $1.5 \pm 0.35 \, \mu g/g$
brain tissue. Elimination from the brain is also very rapid. A
rapid uptake of etomidate is also found in lung, kidney, muscle,
heart and spleen. In these tissues maximum levels are reached
within 2 min after injection. A significantly slower uptake of
etomidate is seen in fat, in the testicles and in the stomach.
Levels in these tissues are maximal between 7 and 28 min after
administration. These observations may be explained by the
solubility of etomidate in an acidic medium (stomach) and by the
lipophilic properties of the unionized drug (HEYKANTS, 1974a).
Since the breakdown of etomidate mainly occurs in the liver (see
below), the concentration of the metabolite in this organ is
higher than that of etomidate, even 3 min after administration.

The distribution of both optical isomers of etomidate (R-(+) and
S-(-)) does not differ substantially in blood, brain and liver.
In spite of almost equal brain concentrations for both isomers,
the S-(+)form has considerably less hypnotic activity, suggesting
the presence of a stereo-specific receptor for etomidate in the
brain (HEYKANTS, 1975).

Etomidate is rapidly metabolized, mainly in the liver, by hydrolysis of the ester group whereby the carboxylic acid of etomidate, which is the main metabolite, is formed. Smaller amounts, provided by lower doses are metabolized more rapidly than larger amounts, provided by higher doses. The metabolite is pharmacologically inactive (HEYKANTS, 1974 a). In rats approx. 78 % (HEYKANTS, 1974a) and in humans approx. 75 % (HEYKANTS et al., 1973) of the intravenously injected dose is excreted with the urine during the first 24 hours after the administration, mainly as the metabolite. Over the same period of time about 13 % of the administered dose is found in the faeces.

In vitro Pharmacology

In in vitro studies etomidate, 2.5 mg/l, was found to have no effect on the Ca^{2+} response-curves in papillary muscles isolated from cats. Besides a weak anti-nicotinic activity no anti-spasmogenic action is produced by etomidate on such tissues as guinea-pig ileum, rabbit duodenum, rabbit spleen and rat fundus (VAN NUETEN, 1974). Yet no overt effect of the hypnotic was observed on the vasoconstriction in isolated peripheral arteries induced by KCl or sympathetic stimulation.

In studies involving intracellular microelectrode techniques, etomidate, 2.5 mg/l, was found to be devoid of any effect on the electrophysiological variables determined in Purkinje fibres and papillary muscles isolated from dog hearts and in papillary and auricular muscles isolated from guinea-pig hearts. Methohexital, 10 mg/l, and propanidid, 50 mg/l, have no significant effect on the variables determined in papillary muscles, but significantly reduce the amplitude and the rate of rise of the action potential and the conduction velocity, and significantly prolong the effective refractory period in Purkinje fibres isolated from dog hearts. In addition, propanidid significantly decreases the spontaneous activity in guinea-pig auricles. These findings demonstrate that at comparative doses, selected on the basis of sleep duration (JAGENEAU et al., 1973), methohexital and propanidid depress the fast sodium conductance in Purkinje fibres, while etomidate is devoid of this side effect (XHONNEUX et al., 1974).

Cardiovascular Pharmacology in Dogs

Experiments on unpremedicated, non-anaesthetized labradors reveal that the cardiovascular effects of etomidate, 1.25 and 2.5 mg/kg i.v., are minimal as compared with those of methohexital, 10 mg/kg i.v., and propanidid, 50 mg/kg i.v. (RENEMAN et al., 1974). In this study comparative doses of the various hypnotics are selected on the basis of sleep duration (JAGENEAU et al., 1973).
The doses of etomidate, methohexital and propanidid, required for adequate sleep durations, are respectively about 5, 6 and 10 times higher in dogs than in man.

At 1.25 mg/kg i.v., etomidate slightly but significantly decreases systolic and diastolic aortic blood pressure, while at 2.5 mg/kg i.v.

this decrease in aortic blood pressure is associated with a slight but significant increase in heart rate. The decrease in aortic blood pressure probably results from a direct vasodilatory property of the compound and the increase in heart rate is likely to be secondary to the decrease in aortic blood pressure since etomidate has no effect on the spontaneous activity in auricular muscle. Etomidate, 1.25 and 2.5 mg/kg i.v., has no significant effect on the maximum first derivative of left ventricular pressure, at constant heart rate, and on mean aortic and mean coronary blood flow.

On the contrary, methohexital, 1o mg/kg i.v., markedly increases heart rate and systolic and diastolic aortic blood pressure and, therefore, the oxygen demand of the left ventricle, while the changes in the maximum first derivative of left ventricular pressure indicate that this hypnotic has some negative inotropic properties (RENEMAN et al., 1974).

Propanidid, 50 mg/kg i.v., has shown to have pronounced negative inotropic properties in this study, as demonstrated by the marked decrease in the maximum first derivative of left ventricular pressure and mean aortic blood flow, in the presence of a pronounced increase in heart rate. Systolic and diastolic blood pressure also decrease after intravenous injection of propanidid.

At doses of 1.25 and 2.5 mg/kg i.v., etomidate does not induce histamine release in unpremedicated, non-anaesthetized beagles. A significant increase in plasma histamine levels, however, is found after intravenous injection of propanidid, 50 mg/kg. An increase, which is not seen after injection of Cremophor, the solvent of propanidid (LADURON and JANSSEN, 1975).

References

1.   HEYKANTS, J.: The distribution, metabolism and excretion of etomidate in the rat. Biological Research Report R 26 490/5. Beerse, Belgium: Janssen Research Products Information Service, 1974 a.

2.   HEYKANTS, J.: The distribution, metabolism and excretion of etomidate in the rat. Comparative pharmacokinetic study of the two optical isomers of etomidate. Biological Research Report R 26 490/7-R 16 333. Beerse, Belgium: Janssen Research Products Information Service, 1974 b.

3.   HEYKANTS, J., BRUGMANS, J., DOENICKE, A.: On the pharmacokinetics of etomidate (R 26 490) in human volunteers: plasma levels, metabolism and excretion. Clinical Research Report R 26 490/1. Beerse, Belgium: Janssen Research Products Information Service, 1973.

4.   JAGENEAU, A.H.M., XHONNEUX, R., RENEMAN, R.S.: Cardiovascular effects of the intravenously injected short-acting hypnotics etomidate, methohexital and propanidid in unanaesthetized dogs. Biological Research Report R 26 490/3. Beerse, Belgium: Janssen Research Products Information Service, 1973.

5. JANSSEN, P.A.J., NIEMEGEERS, C.J.E., MARSBOOM, R.P.H.: Etomidate, a potent non-barbiturate hypnotic. Intravenous etomidate in mice, rats, guinea-pigs, rabbits and dogs. Archives Internationales de Pharmacodynamie et de Therapie 214 (1), P. 92-132 (1975).

6. JANSSEN, P.A.J., NIEMEGEERS, C.J.E., SCHELLEKENS, K.H.L., LENAERTS, F.M.: Etomidate, R-(+)-ethyl-1 (∝-methyl-benzyl)imidazole-5-carboxylate (R 16 659), a potent, short-acting and relatively atoxic intravenous hypnotic agent in rats. Arzneimittel-Forsch.: 21, 1234-1243 (1971).

7. LADURON, P., JANSSEN, P.A.J.: Histamine release in dogs after intravenous injection of etomidate. Biological Research Report R 26 490/1. Beerse, Belgium: Janssen Research Products Information Service, 1973.

8. MEULDERMANS, W., HEYKANTS, J.: The plasma protein binding and distribution of etomidate in dog, rat and human blood. A comparative study between commonly used methods for the determination of protein-drug interaction. Archives Internationales de Pharmacodynamic et de Therapie 221, P. 150-162 (1976).

9. RENEMAN, R.S., JAGENEAU, A.H.M., XHONNEUX, R., LADURON, P.: The cardiovascular pharmacology of etomidate (R 26 490), a new, potent and short-acting intravenous hypnotic agent. Proceedings 4th Europ. Congress of Anaesthesiology, Madrid 1974. Amsterdam-London: Excerpta Medica Congress Series, 347, P. 152-156.

10. VAN NUETEN, J.M.: Etomidate, a short-acting non-barbiturate hypnotic. Study on cardiac tissues and on smooth muscle preparations in vitro. Biological Research Report R 26 490/6. Beerse, Belgium: Janssen Research Products Information Service, 1974.

11. XHONNEUX, R., CARMELIET, E., RENEMAN, R.S.: The electrophysiological effects of etomidate (R 26 490), a new, short-acting hypnotic, in various cardiac tissues. Proceedings 4th Europ. Congress of Anaesthesiology, Madrid 1974. Amsterdam-London: Excerpta Medica Congress Series, 347, P. 157-161.

Protein Binding of Etomidate

G.A. Mannes and A. Doenicke

The Method

The etomidate binding to human albumin (50 g/l) was ascertained by means of the equilibrium dialysis. The walls of the dialysing membrane were 0.02 mm thick with a mean porewidth of 2.4 mm. Using a dialysing temperature of $2^{\circ}C$, a balance between internal and external fluid was obtained after 8 hours.
The percentage of protein-bound etomidate is calculated with the aid of the following formula:

$$EPB = 100 \text{ \%} \frac{c_2 - c_1}{c_2}$$

c_1 = concentration of etomidate in the protein-free external fluid, which is in balance with the concentration of unbound etomidate in the plasma water of the internal fluid.
c_2 = concentration of etomidate in the internal fluid.

Tritium-labelled etomidate was at our disposal for the experiments. We used permablend III by Packard Instruments as a solvent, which was diluted with toluene according to instructions.

Results

With a pH of 7.4 the etomidate binding to human albumin amounts to 64.89 ± 3.74 %. The binding is pH-dependent: with pH 6.0 the binding value is 61.48 ± 4.79; with pH 3.5 it only amounts to 26.78 ± 3.06 %.

Discussion

The protein binding of a drug is an unspecific reversible reaction via hydrophobus interactions, ionic bond (GOLDSTEIN et al., 1968) and hydrogen bridge linkage. Only the free and unbound part has a pharmacological effect. If the free part is diminished, the bound part dissociates again, thereby becoming again pharmacologically effective.

The etomidate binding can well be compared with that of thiopentone, 65.3 ± 0.7 % of which is bound to human albumin under comparable conditions. 88.1 ± 0.4 % of thiopentone is bound to human plasma and 91.2 % to whole blood (MANNES and DOENICKE, 1975).

Although the result of the protein binding of etomidate to human albumin will have to be completed by further experiments with plasma, haemoglobin, and muscular protein, one may assume that etomidate is bound to plasma proteins in a similarly high degree as thiopentone. The binding of a drug to plasma proteins is a relevant factor for the process of distribution in the organism. With the so-called shot-injection the initial concentrations are higher than with a slow injection of the same dosage. The protein binding depends on the concentration; with increasing concentrations the free part increases exponentially. Since only the free part can leave the vascular system and diffuse into the tissue, the distribution process in the organism will be quite different with a shot-injection (DOST, 1968; KURZ, 1969; MANNES and DOENICKE, 1975).
The occurence of an acidosis may lead to an intensification of the hypnotic effects by increasing the free part in the blood (KURZ and MOHR, 1968). By treating the acidosis with alkaline valences, the narcotic effect is decreasing, because with a higher pH the etomidate binding to plasma proteins increases.

Summary

With a pH of 7.4 about 65 % of etomidate is bound to human albumin; thiopentone is known to possess a similar high binding rate. It is assumed that the protein binding value reached by etomidate with human plasma is similar to that of thiopentone, in the order of about 88 %.

Not only the clinical experiments, e.g. EEG controls of reinjections of etomidate (DOENICKE et al., KUGLER and DOENICKE, 1975), but also clinical observations led to suppose that the protein binding of etomidate was of clinical interest.
Within the scope of a major study of the protein binding of thiopentone under different conditions (change of temperature, acid- and basedisplacement) we also included etomidate in this study in 1973.

Zusammenfassung

Etomidate wird bei einem pH von 7,4 zu ca. 65 % an Humanalbumin gebunden; eine ähnlich hohe Bindungsrate ist auch von Thiopental bekannt. Es wird angenommen, daß Etomidate an Humanplasma einen Proteinbindungswert ähnlich Thiopental mit ca. 88 % erreicht.

References

1. DOENICKE, A., KUGLER, J., PENZEL, G., LAUB, M., KALMAR, L., KILLIAN, J., BEZECNY, H.: Hirnfunktion und Toleranzbreite nach Etomidate, einem neuen barbituratfreien i.v. applizierbaren Hypnotikum. Anaesthesist _22_, 357 (1973).

2. DOST, F.H.: Grundlagen der Pharmakokinetik, S. 195 Stuttgart 1968.

8

3. GOLDSTEIN, A., ARONOW, A., KALMAN, S.H.: Principles of drug action.
    New York-Evanston-London: Harper & Row 1968.

4. KUGLER, J., DOENICKE, A.: EEG and Etomidate. Anaesthesiologie und Wieder-
    belebung, Bd. 106. Berlin-Heidelberg-New York: Springer.

5. KURZ, H.: Einfluß der Proteinbindung auf die Verteilung von Arzneimitteln
    nach schneller und langsamer Injektion. Arch.Pharmak.exp.Path. 263,
    233 (1969).

6. KURZ, A.A., MOHR, E.: Der Einfluß von Acidose und Alkalose auf die Bin-
    dung von Arzneimitteln an Plasmaproteine. Arch.Pharmak.exp.Path. 260,
    164 (1968).

7. MANNES, G.A., DOENICKE, A.: Thiopental, eine pharmakologische Studie.
    Anaesthesist, im Druck.

THE EFFECT OF INTRA-ARTERIAL INJECTION OF ETOMIDATE AND THIOPENTAL ON THE SKELETAL MUSCLE- AND ARTERIAL WALL-STRUCTURES

R.S. Reneman, F. Verheyen, R. Kruger, W. van Gerven and M. Borges

Introduction

In the clinic, the consequences of an accidental intra-arterial injection of thiopental are well known. They range from gangrene and ischaemic contracture of muscles in the severe cases to minor degrees of anaesthesia of digits in the more fortunate patient (KINMONTH and SHEPHARD, 1959). It is rather likely that these disturbances mainly result from direct arterial damage and thrombosis (COHEN, 1948a and 1948b; STONE and DONNELLY, 1961) since arterial vasoconstriction, if present, during or after the injection of thiopental is only temporary and arterial spasm has never been demonstrated (KINMONTH and SHEPHERD, 1959; BURN and HOBBS, 1959; BURN, 1960).

The present study was conducted to investigate the effects, if any, of intra-arterial injection of etomidate on the structures of skeletal muscle and arteries. Thiopental served as a reference substance, and was injected intra-arterially in separate experiments.

Methods

1. Experimental Set-up

The experiments were performed on 15 rabbits of the New-Zealand strain of varying age and sex, and ranging in weight between 2200 and 3500 g (mean 2933 g). The animals were premedicated with Hypnorm, 1 mg/kg i.m., and the femoral artery was dissected free for injection of etomidate or thiopental. The hypnotics were carefully injected into the artery through a fine, short (9 mm) needle (26 G) inserted just below the inguinal ligament. The needle-point was directed in a distal direction. Both etomidate and thiopental were injected over a period of one minute.

The rabbits were divided into three groups of 5 animals each. In the first group (group I) etomidate was injected into the left femoral artery and distilled water into the right one. In this group, the animals were premedicated again with Hypnorm 20 - 25 hours after injection of the hypnotic, and the anterior tibial muscle and the extensor digitorum longus muscle were completely removed from both the left and the right hind-leg without touching

the muscle with forceps or scissors. At the site of injection of
the hypnotic, the femoral artery was opened and checked on patency,
and the vessel wall was examined macroscopically for damage. In
the second group (group II), etomidate was injected into the left
femoral artery. The rabbits were premedicated again with Hypnorm
7 days after the injection of the hypnotic, and the anterior tibial
muscle and the extensor digitorum longus muscle were removed from
the left hind-leg, and the left femoral artery was inspected at the
site of injection as above mentioned. In this group a segment of
the femoral artery, 1-2 cm distal to the site of injection, was
also removed. In the third group (group III) thiopental was injected into the left femoral artery, and the same procedure was followed as in the second group.

2. *Compounds*

Etomidate-sulphate was dissolved in 1.8 mg $Na_2 HPO_4 \cdot 12 H_2O$ and
2.2 mg $NaH_2PO_4 \cdot H_2O$ with 4.2 % glucose in the clinically used
concentration of 1.5 mg etomidate-base/ml (pH = about 3.4).
At each intra-arterial injection 2.5 mg/kg was given.

Thiopental sodium (Nesdonal) was dissolved in distilled water in
a concentration of 100 mg/ml. Thiopental was injected intra-
arterially at a dose of 15 mg/kg.

3. *Histology*

After excision, the muscles were rinsed and carefully sliced
transversely into pieces of approx. 2 mm thickness. Comparable
samples were taken from the proximal, the middle and the distal
part of the muscles and were fixed in 4 % formaldehyde for
3 - 7 days. The femoral artery samples in the second and the third
group were also sliced in segments of approx. 2 mm and prepared
in the same way as the muscle samples.

After fixation, the tissue samples were further dehydrated in
graded series of ethanol, cleared in xylene and routinely em-
bedded in paraffin. Sections of 5 μm thickness were prepared and
stained with hematoxylin-eosin and Weigert-Van Gieson's stain.
The sections were examined with a Leitz light-microscope.

Results

At macroscopical examination all the femoral arteries looked
normal at the site of injection. In one case of group II, the
patency of the artery could not be checked because the animal
died after receiving its premedication. The other femoral arteries
were patent.

In group I, no histological changes could be detected, neither in
the muscle itself nor in the intramuscular arteries, 20 - 24
hours after injection of etomidate or distilled water.

In group II, 2 of the 5 arterial segments taken 1 - 2 cm distal
to the site of injection, showed some intimal thickening 7 days
after injection of etomidate. The muscles looked normal, i.e.
clear cross-striation of the contractile elements and normal
peripherally located nuclei (Fig. 1). Infiltration of polymorphonuclear leucocytes of any importance was not observed.
The intramuscular arteries were not constricted and did not
reveal histological changes (Fig. 2).

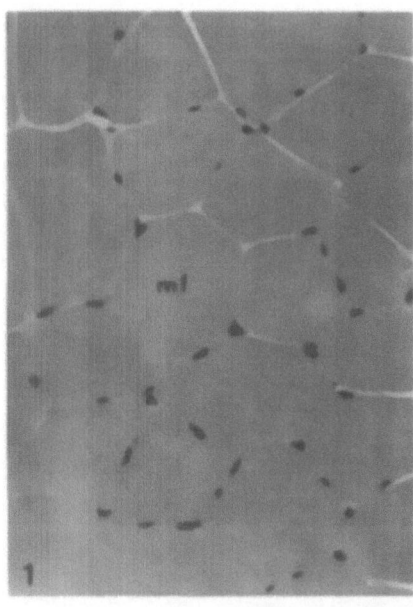

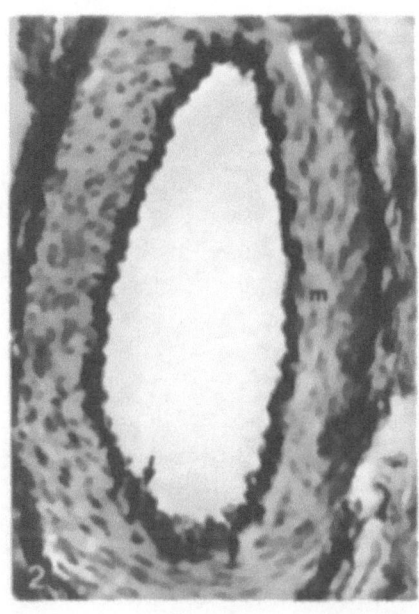

*Fig. 1.Intra-arterial injection of
etomidate (2.5 mg/kg). Normal muscle
fibres (mf), with peripherally
located nuclei, of the extensor
digitorum longus muscle are shown.
(X 300)*

*Fig. 2.Intra-arterial injection of
etomidate (2.5 mg/kg). Transverse
section of a normally structured intramuscular artery. No intimal proliferation is observed. The arrow points to
the internal elastic lamina. m = media
(X 275)*

The arterial segments, 1 - 2 cm distal to the site of injection,
showed similar intimal changes in group III as in group II; in
two arteries the intima was thickened 7 days after the injection
of thiopental. All the muscles in this group showed extensive
areas of necrosis as demonstrated by swelling and dislocation of
the nuclei, the loss of cross-striation and the intensive staining
with eosin. Occasionally infiltration of polymorphonuclear
leucocytes, especially eosinophylic ones, was found in the muscles
of one rabbit. Invasion of fibroblasts and formation of scar
tissue was seen in several clearly defined areas (Fig. 3). The
necrosis and fibrosis in the anterior tibial muscle and the

extensor digitorum longus muscle was usually more pronounced in
the distal than in the proximal parts. Several intramuscular
arteries showed extensive intimal proliferation and intimal
oedema (Fig. 4). Some of these arteries were completely occluded.
In the severely affected areas some arteries showed medial lesions
with infiltration of polymorphonuclear leucocytes and erythrocytes.
The histologically unchanged small arteries and arterioles in the
muscles were not constricted.

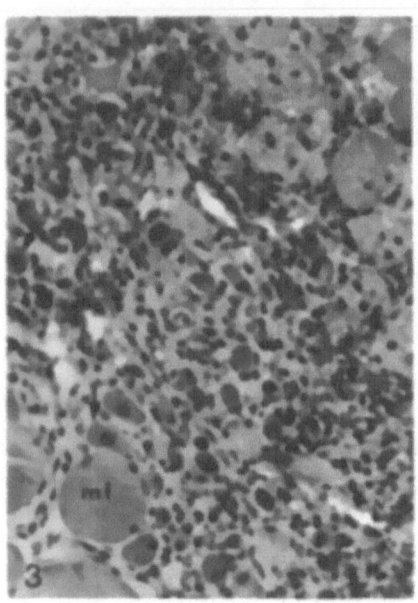

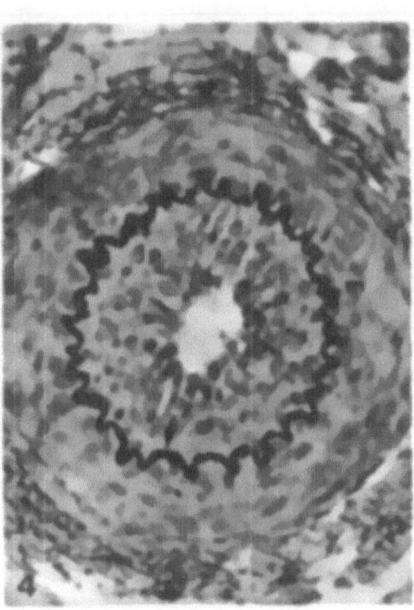

Fig. 3.*Intra-arterial injection of
thiopental (15 mg/kg). Remnants of
muscle fibres with centrally located
nuclei (arrows) are surrounded by
invaded fibroblasts. Some rounded
fibres (mf) of approx. normal size
are seen at the upper right.
(X 300)*

Fig. 4.*Intra-arterial injection of thiopental (15 mg/kg). The extensive intimal
proliferation (ip) and intimal oedema of
this intramuscular artery is apparent.
The arrow points to the internal elastic
lamina. m = media (X 400)*

Discussion

The present study shows that in rabbits injection of thiopental
into the femoral artery leads to necrosis and fibrosis in the
anterior tibial muscle and the extensor digitorum longus muscle,
and to intimal proliferation and intimal oedema in the intramuscular arteries. In several of these arteries, the proliferation
and oedema resulted in total occlusion of the vessel. The
unaffected arteries were not constricted. Etomidate is devoid of
these serious side-effects.

The tissue necrosis seen after the intra-arterial injection of thiopental is in accordance with the findings of such investigators as COHEN (1948a), KINMONTH and SHEPHERD (1959), and BURNS (1960). Our study supports the idea of COHEN (1948a, b) and KINMONTH and SHEPHERD (1959), that the essential pathology of intra-arterial thiopental is not arterial spasm, but intense intimal damage of the arteries. The thrombosis in the affected arteries after intra-arterial injection of thiopental in humans (COHEN, 1948b), was not found in rabbits. These diverse findings might be the result of differences in the thrombogenesis in the two species.

In this study we have chosen for injection into the femoral artery rather than into one of the ear arteries, because we wanted to study the effect of intra-arterial etomidate on skeletal muscle and because the anterior tibial muscle is known to be susceptible to arterial lesions (RENEMAN, 1968). The more pronounced necrosis and fibrosis in the distal parts of the anterior tibial muscle and the extensor digitorum longus muscle after intra-arterial thiopental can be explained by the higher vulnerability of these muscle parts in case of disturbances in the arterial blood supply (LE GROS CLARK, 1946).

The fact that intra-arterial injection of etomidate, at a dose level 5 - 6 times higher than the clinical dose, is devoid of any significant effect on the structures of skeletal muscle and arteries, in a model which has shown to be sensitive to intra-arterial injections of thiopental, demonstrates that also in this respect etomidate can be considered a safe hypnotic.

Acknowledgements

The authors are indebted to Lambert Leyssen for taking the photographs and to Christiane Van den Broeck for technical assistance.

Summary

In this study the effect of intra-arterial injection of etomidate and thiopental on the structures of skeletal muscle and arterial wall was studied in rabbits. Intra-arterial thiopental leads to necrosis and fibrosis in skeletal muscle and to intimal proliferation and intimal oedema in the intramuscular arteries. In several of these arteries, the proliferation and oedema resulted in total occlusion of the vessel. Etomidate was devoid of these serious side-effects.

Zusammenfassung

In diesem Versuch werden die Effekte von intraarteriell injiziertem Etomidate und Thiopental auf die Strukturen des Skelettmuskels und der Arterienwand bei Kaninchen untersucht. Intraarterielles Thiopental führt zu Nekrose und Fibrose im Skelettmuskel und zu Intimaproliferation und Ödem in den intramuskulären Arterien.

In verschiedenen dieser Arterien entstand infolge der Proliferation und Ödeme eine völlige Gefäßverödung. Bei Etomidate kamen diese schweren Nebenwirkungen nicht vor.

References

1. BURN, J.H.: Why thiopentone injected into an artery may cause gangrene. Brit.med.J. 1960 II, 414.

2. BURN, J.H., HOBBS, R.: Mechanism of arterial spasm following intra-arterial injection of thiopentone. Lancet 1959 I, 1112.

3. COHEN, S.M.: Accidental intra-arterial injection of drugs. Lancet 1948a II, 361.

4. COHEN, S.M.: Accidental intra-arterial injection of drugs. Lancet 1948b II, 409.

5. KINMONTH, J.B., SHEPHERD, R.C.: Accidental injection of thiopentone into artery. Studies of pathology and treatment. Brit.med.J. 1959 II, 914.

6. LE GROS CLARK, W.E.: An experimental study of the regeneration of mammalian striped muscle. Anatomy 80 (1946).

7. RENEMAN, R.S.: The anterior and lateral compartment syndrome of the leg. The Hague-Paris: Mouton, 1968.

8. STONE, H.H., DONNELLY, C.C.: The accidental intra-arterial injection of thiopental. Anaesthesiology 22, 995 (1961).

Interaction between Etomidate and the Antihypertensive Agents Propranolol and α-Methyl-Dopa

R.S. Reneman, W. Van Gerven and R. Kruger

Introduction

Anti-hypertensive treatment is fairly common in patients who are
subject to surgical procedures. Since some anti-hypertensive
agents are known to potentiate the hypotensive effects of anaesthetics and hypnotics (STUMP and FLEMING, 1965, KIENLEN, 1974)
and since etomidate slightly but significantly decreases arterial
blood pressure (RENEMAN et al., in press), the present study was
conducted to investigate the interference, if any, of etomidate
with propranolol and α-methyl-dopa in unanaesthetized dogs.

Methods

The experiments were performed on 12 unpremedicated, non-anaesthetized labradors of either sex and varying age, ranging in
weight between 20 and 35 kg (median: 25 kg). The animals were
trained to lie down quietly for the duration of the experiment.

The ECG was derived from limb leads. Heart rate was counted from
the ECG. Ascending aortic pressure was measured in mmHg through
a silastic catheter connected to a pressure transducer (TELCO).
The catheter was implanted directly in the aorta, at least 5 days
prior to the experiments. Respiratory rate was assessed by
counting the number of respirations per minute with a stopwatch.
The sleep duration was also determined. Opening of the eyes,
usually accompanied by raising of the head, was regarded as the
end of sleep. Only stage V and VI of MAGNUS-GIRNDT were accepted
as adequate sleep (stage V = anaesthesia, cornea- and eyelid
reflex present; stage VI = anaesthesia, no reflexes present).
Before each experiment a catheter was inserted into a fore- or
hindleg vein for the injection of etomidate. The ECG and the
analogue pressure signal were recorded continuously on a multi-
channel SCHWARZER recorder.

The animals were divided into two groups of 6 animals each. In the
first group the effects of intravenous injections of etomidate,
2.5 mg/kg, were studied both before and after treatment with
propranolol (Inderal). Propranolol was administered orally at a
dose of 10 mg/kg for three days. In the second group these effects
were studied before and after oral treatment with α-methyl-dopa
(Aldomet) at a dose of 100 mg/kg for three days. Treatment with
propranolol and α-methyl-dopa started 2 days after the first
injection of etomidate. In both groups the second etomidate
injection was given 2-4 hours after the last administration of
the anti-hypertensive drug.

Table 1. The effect of etomidate (2.5 mg/kg i.v.) on heart rate (beats/min), systolic and diastolic aortic blood pressure (mmHg) and respiratory rate (breaths/min) before and after treatment with propranolol (10 mg/kg orally) for three days in unanaesthetized labradors (n = 6)

Variables	Before etomidate		After etomidate					
	- 15'	0	1'	2.5'	5'	7.5'	10'	15'
Heart Rate								
Before								
median	132.5	120	125	117.5	110	97.5	115	102.5
95 % limits	80 – 155	85 – 150	100 – 155	80 – 150	80 – 135	90 – 130	90 – 130	80 – 170
After								
median	90*	100*	105	97.5	90	87.5	87.5	97.5
95 % limits	60 – 120	60 – 120	90 – 120	60 – 120	70 – 120	70 – 105	60 – 105	60 – 105
P		NS+	NS‡	NS‡	NS‡	NS‡	NS‡	NS‡
Systolic Aortic Pressure								
Before								
median	132.5	137.5	125	112.5	112.5	112.5	125	132.5
95 % limits	120 – 175	110 – 170	105 – 135	105 – 135	100 – 135	100 – 140	110 – 145	115 – 140
After								
median	125	122.5	112.5	107.5	105	105	105	107.5
95 % limits	120 – 150	120 – 150	95 – 170	105 – 160	100 – 155	100 – 150	100 – 140	95 – 155
P		NS	NS	NS	NS	NS	NS	NS
Diastolic Aortic Pressure								
Before								
median	80	82.5	80	70	75	72.5	80	82.5
95 % limits	60 – 110	60 – 115	50 – 90	50 – 85	55 – 90	55 – 100	55 – 100	60 – 95
After								
median	72.5	72.5	62.5	62.5	57.5	57.5	62.5	62.5
95 % limits	60 – 90	65 – 95	55 – 130	45 – 120	40 – 110	45 – 105	55 – 85	55 – 90
P		NS	NS	NS	NS	NS	NS	NS

Respiratory Rate

Before	median	28	28	30	36	40	42	45	42
	95 % limits	18 – 60	20 – 68	16 – 44	18 – 42	18 – 52	19 – 60	20 – 96	21 – 48
After	median	28	28	20	24	24	28	28	28
	95 % limits	20 – 64	20 – 72	18 – 32	20 – 30	20 – 32	20 – 42	24 – 46	24 – 42
	P	NS	NS	NS	NS	NS	NS	NS	NS

* significantly lower than before treatment with propranolol ($P < 0.05$).

\+ comparison of the differences between the values before and after propranolol just before injection with those 15 min before injection of etomidate.

\# comparison of the differences between the values before and after propranolol at different intervals after injection with those just before (0) injection of etomidate.

Table 2. The effect of etomidate (2.5 mg/kg i.v.) on heart rate (beats/min), systolic and diastolic aortic blood pressure (mmHg) and respiratory rate (breaths/min) before and after treatment with α-methyl-dopa (100 mg/kg orally) for three days in unanaesthetized labradors (n = 6)

Variables		Before etomidate		After etomidate					
		– 15'	0	1'	2.5'	5'	7.5'	10'	15'
Heart Rate									
Before	median	115	110	120	105	95	95	100	110
	95 % limits	100 – 120	100 – 120	100 – 130	80 – 120	70 – 110	75 – 100	85 – 120	80 – 120
After	median	105	105	115	105	105	97.5	100	110
	95 % limits	90 – 140	80 – 120	70 – 120	65 – 120	65 – 120	70 – 120	75 – 120	75 – 130
	P		NS+	NS‡	NS‡	NS‡	NS‡	NS‡	NS‡
Systolic Aortic Pressure									
Before	median	137.5	132.5	140	135	125	130	132.5	147.5
	95 % limits	120 – 185	120 – 180	110 – 160	110 – 150	105 – 160	100 – 160	110 – 175	120 – 180
After	median	107.5*	102.5*	107.5	105	100	100	105	110
	95 % limits	95 – 115	90 – 110	80 – 135	80 – 125	80 – 120	80 – 110	90 – 115	90 – 115
	P		NS	NS	NS	NS	NS	NS	NS
Diastolic Aortic Pressure									
Before	median	90	87.5	95	80	77.5	80	85	100
	95 % limits	70 – 120	70 – 100	70 – 120	70 – 110	70 – 110	70 – 105	70 – 110	80 – 125
After	median	67.5*	62.5*	72.5	65	62.5	62.5	67.5	70
	95 % limits	55 – 80	55 – 80	35 – 105	45 – 100	50 – 90	50 – 80	50 – 85	55 – 80
	P		NS	NS	NS	NS	NS	NS	NS

Respiratory Rate

Before								
median	26	27	29.5	26	30	31	33.5	29
95 % limits	24 – 30	24 – 32	12 – 40	22 – 44	22 – 48	22 – 46	24 – 48	24 – 40
After								
median	20*	17*	19	20	26	23	21	22
95 % limits	12 – 28	9 – 28	6 – 28	12 – 40	13 – 40	12 – 40	14 – 40	14 – 48
P	NS	NS	NS	NS	NS	NS	NS	NS

* significantly lower than before treatment with α—methyl-dopa (P < 0.05)

+ comparison of the differences between the values before and after α—methyl-dopa just before injection with those 15 min before injection of etomidate.

comparison of the differences between the values before and after α—methyl-dopa at different intervals after injection with those just before (O) injection of etomidate.

Etomidate-sulphate was dissolved in 1.8 mg $Na_2HPO_4 \cdot 12$ aqua and 2.2 mg $NaH_2PO_4 \cdot 1$ aqua with 4.2 % glucose in a concentration of 1.5 mg base/ml (pH = 3.4). After a recorded control period of 30 min, the hypnotic was injected through the intravenous catheter over a period of approx. 30 sec. The variables were determined 15 min and just before and 1, 2.5, 5, 7.5, 10 and 15 min after the injection. The heart rate and blood pressure values represent an average determined over 10 heart beats.

Changes in the values of the determined variables after three days of treatment with propranolol or α-methyl-dopa, compared with the values two days before compound administration were evaluated for statistical significance using WILCOXON's matched-pairs signed-ranks test (two-tailed probability). Differences between the values of the determined variables before and after treatment with the anti-hypertensive drugs at various intervals before and after the injection of etomidate were compared with each other and evaluated for statistical significance also by applying WILCOXON's test (two-tailed probability).

Results

After three days of oral treatment, propanolol, 10 mg/kg per day, significantly decreased heart rate, but had no significant effect on systolic and diastolic aortic blood pressure and respiratory rate (Table 1). α-methyl-dopa, 100 mg/kg orally per day for three days, significantly decreased systolic and diastolic aortic blood pressure and respiratory rate. No significant changes were found in heart rate after the administration of α-methyl-dopa (Table 2).

Since the differences between the values of the determined variables before and after treatment with propranolol or α-methyl-dopa 15 min before the injection of etomidate were not significantly different from those just before the injection, the latter differences were used as control values for comparison with the differences between the values of the variables before and after administration of the anti-hypertensive agents at the various intervals after injection of the hypnotic. In none of the determined variables, significant changes could be detected in these differences after intravenous injection of etomidate, 2.5 mg/kg i.v., compared with the differences just before administration of the hypnotic (Table 1 and 2).

After treatment with either propranolol or α-methyl-dopa, the duration of sleep induced by 2.5 mg/kg etomidate i.v. was not significantly different from that before anti-hypertensive treatment (Table 3).

Discussion

In unanaesthetized labradors intravenous injection of etomidate slightly, but significantly decreases systolic and diastolic aortic blood pressure and slightly increases heart rate (RENEMAN et al., in print). The present study shows that these effects

Table 3. The duration of sleep induced by etomidate (2.5 mg/kg i.v.) before and after oral treatment with propranolol (10 mg/kg) or $\propto$-methyl-dopa (100 mg/kg) for three days in unanaesthetized labradors

| | | Duration of Sleep | |
		Before	After
Propranolol (n = 6)			
	median :	10'	10' [+]
	95 % limits :	7.5' - 10'	10' - 16'
$\propto$methyl-dopa (n = 6)			
	median :	8'45"	10' [+]
	95 % limits :	5' - 10'	10' - 20'

[+] P > 0.05

are not potentiated by oral pretreatment with the anti-hypertensive agents propranolol and $\propto$-methyl-dopa. Yet the decrease in heart rate and in respiratory rate seen after the administration of propranolol and $\propto$-methyl-dopa, respectively, are not significantly affected by the injection of etomidate. The absence of a significant depressor effect of propranolol in unanaesthetized normotensive dogs is in accordance with the finding of HALKOLA et al. (1974), who injected propranolol intravenously.

Chlorpromazine and reserpine prolong the duration of sleep induced by pentobarbital (MALHOTRA, 1962), and $\propto$-methyl-dopa that induced by methohexital and hexobarbital (KIENLEN, 1974). In our study both propranolol and $\propto$-methyl-dopa had no significant effect on the duration of sleep induced by intravenous injection of etomidate. The doses of etomidate required for adequate sleep durations are approx. 5-times higher in dogs than in man, which is also known for other hypnotics as methohexital (6-times higher) and propanidid (10-times higher) (JAGENEAU et al., 1973).

In conclusion one can say that in the present study the anti-hypertensive agents propranolol and $\propto$-methyl-dopa do not interfere with the action of etomidate, at least as far as the effect on heart rate, aortic blood pressure, respiratory rate and duration of sleep is concerned.

Acknowledgement

The authors are indebted to Mr. J. Dony for his help in the statistical evaluation of the results and to Mr. J. Lambregts for his technical assistance.

Summary

In this study the interaction between the anti-hypertensive agents propranolol and α-methyl-dopa and etomidate was studied in unpremedicated, non-anaesthetized labradors. No interference was found between these anti-hypertensive drugs and etomidate, at least as far as the effect on heart rate, systolic and diastolic aortic blood pressure, respiratory rate and duration of sleep is concerned.

Zusammenfassung

In diesem Versuch wird die Wechselwirkung zwischen den antihypertensiven Mitteln Propranolol, α-Methyldopa und Etomidate an nicht vorbehandelten und nicht anästhesierten Labrador-Hunden geprüft. Es wurde zwischen beiden blutdrucksenkenden Mitteln und Etomidate in Hinsicht auf Herzfrequenz, systolischen und diastolischen aortischen Blutdruck, Atemfrequenz und Schlafdauer keine Interferenz festgestellt.

References

1. HALKOLA, L., KOIVIKKO, A., LÄNSIMIES, E.: Hemodynamic effects of chloralose and propranolol in dogs. Acta physiol. scand. 90, 505-508 (1974).

2. JAGENEAU, A.H.M., XHONNEUX, R., RENEMAN, R.S.: Cardiovascular effects of the intravenously injected short-acting hypnotics etomidate, methohexital and propanidid in unanaesthetized dogs. Biological Research Report R 26490/3. Beerse, Belgium: Janssen Research Products Information Service, 1973.

3. KIENLEN, J.: Interférences des médicaments de l'hypertension arterielle avec l'anesthésie (en dehors des beta bloquants). Ann. Anesth. franc. 15, 45-60 (1974).

4. MALHOTRA, C.L., DAS, P.K., DHALLA, N.S.: Investigations on the mechanism of potentiation of barbiturate hypnosis by hersaponin, acorus oil, reserpine and chlorpromazine. Arch. int. Pharmacodyn. 138, 537-547 (1962).

5. RENEMAN, R.S., JAGENEAU, A.H.M., XHONNEUX, R., LADURON, P.: The cardiovascular pharmacology of etomidate (R 26490), a new, potent and short-acting intravenous hypnotic agent. Recent Progress in Anaesthesiology and Resuscitation Publ.: Amsterdam-London: Excerpta Medica 1975.

6. STUMP, J.M., FLEMING, W.W.: The effect of guanethidine, cocaine and reserpine on the hypotensive action of thiopental. J. Pharmacol.exp.Ther. 147, 298-302 (1965).

Teratogenicity of Etomidate[+]

A. Doenicke and M. Haehl

After the accident with thalidomide a very intensive investigation of the teratogenic action of drugs has been started. As we thought the teratogenic damage rate of more than 60 % after halothane as quoted by BASFORD and FINK being rather high, we have checked these results of 1968 in the course of our further experiments and completed them with data on thiopental, propanidid and etomidate.

These are some results: from a comparison of percentages we found clearly less anomalies in vertebrae and ribs after halothane (0.8-Vol %) than did BASFORD and FINK. We ascribe the discrepancy in the results to the higher test temperature (31° C) and to the considerably larger number of foetuses (11.000 in the halothane-nitrous oxide series) (DOENICKE and WITTMANN, 1975).

We have recently pointed at the high abortion rates after halothane (WITTMANN et al., 1974; DOENICKE et al., 1975).

Intravenous anaesthetics, such as thiopental at therapeutic doses of 20 and 40 mg/kg bodyweight in rat, have not been studied so far. With regard to overall anomaly rates, the wistar rat with its 50 % reaches a level comparable to halothane. With 27 % the Sprague-Dawley strain remained clearly below this number. As a rule both strains were especially sensitive on the 9th-11th day of pregnancy, roughly corresponding to the 8th week in man.

Moreover, we were able to make an interesting comparison with barbiturate-free anaesthetics such as propanidid and etomidate.

In the Sprague-Dawley strain, we even found a lower anomaly rate in the etomidate-treated group than in the control animals. With an incidence of 10.2 % the wistar rates, however, being more sensitive to etomidate, exceeded the control value only by 1 %.

A brief comparison with the earlier results showed: thiopental gave rise to an increase in rib anomalies in wistar rats from 20 to 60 %, in the Sprague-dawley strain from about 9 to 18 %.

As compared to an untreated control group, halothane (0.8 %) 1.5 l O_2 / 0.5 l N_2O) increased the rib anomaly rate from 11 to 21 %. Vertebral anomalies after etomidate reached a rate of about 1 %.

[+]Supported by the Minister of Health / Germany

Summary

From the results of these investigations we conclude that barbiturate-free hypnotics - propanidid shows the same favourable characteristics as etomidate - have no teratogenic effects and are even more advantageous than barbiturates during the first months of pregnancy.

Zusammenfassung

Nach diesen Untersuchungen kommen wir zu dem Schluß, daß die barbituratfreien Narkotika - Propanidid verhält sich ähnlich günstig wie Etomidate - keine teratogenen Wirkungen zeigen und somit in den ersten Schwangerschaftsmonaten Vorteile gegenüber den Barbituraten aufweisen.

References

1. BASFORD, A.B., FINK, B.R.: The Teratogenicity of Halothane in the Rat. Anaesthesiologie 29, 1167 61968).

2. DOENICKE, A., WITTMANN, R.: Effet tératogène de L'Halothane sur le Foetus de Rat. Anesth.Analg.Réanim. 32, 47 (1975).

3. DOENICKE, A., WITTMANN, R., HEINRICH, H., PAUSCH, H.: L'Effet abortif de L'Halothane. Anesth.Analg.Réanim. 32, 41 (1975).

4. WITTMANN, R., DOENICKE, A., HEINRICH, H., PAUSCH, H.: Die abortive Wirkung von Halothan. Anaesthesist 23, 3o (1974).

Etomidate, a New Hypnotic Agent for Intravenous Application

A. Doenicke

After successful animal experiments (JANSSEN et al., 1971) we investigated the hypnotic potency and the cardiovascular activity of the new substance etomidate on volunteers.

The main advantage of volunteers in comparison to clinical trials is that consideration of various disturbing effects of illness and surgical intervention can be excluded.

Double-blind studies on hypnotics and narcotics, that have already stood their test in hospitals, help to judge the qualities of the unknown drug (DOENICKE, 1973).

Necessary precautionary measures (EEG and ECG) were done on the patient before this hypnotic was first administered to him on March 21, 1972. Intra-arterial blood pressure, heart rate and respiration were checked constantly. For obvious reasons the dosage selected at that time was low. As a result it was just sufficient to perform only a minor operation on an outpatient. No significant influence on the cardiovascular system or respiration was observed. The EEG showed typical sleeping stages similar to those after barbiturate narcosis. An analysis of data from 25 further unselected patients did not show any major change of the circulatory parameters.

As many narcotics are known to produce an increased histamine release (LORENZ et al., 1972) we were particularly interested in this aspect. Encouraged by the results in the first 25 patients we measured the plasma histamine levels in volunteers after etomidate hypnosis. Blood samples for differential blood smear were collected, control of blood pressure and heart rate was done repeatedly before, during and after the hypnosis.

A comparison with 3 known hypnotics at this stage of the investigation reveals that only etomidate does not release histamine (Fig. 1).

Even the constant level of basophilic leukocytes in the blood, the stability of blood pressure and heart rate, and the absence of erythemas indicated no release of histamine after etomidate administration (DOENICKE et al., 1973).

The initial impressions were confirmed by a subsequent clinical trial which was set up to analyse data on the range of blood pressure after etomidate was given as compared to propanidid.

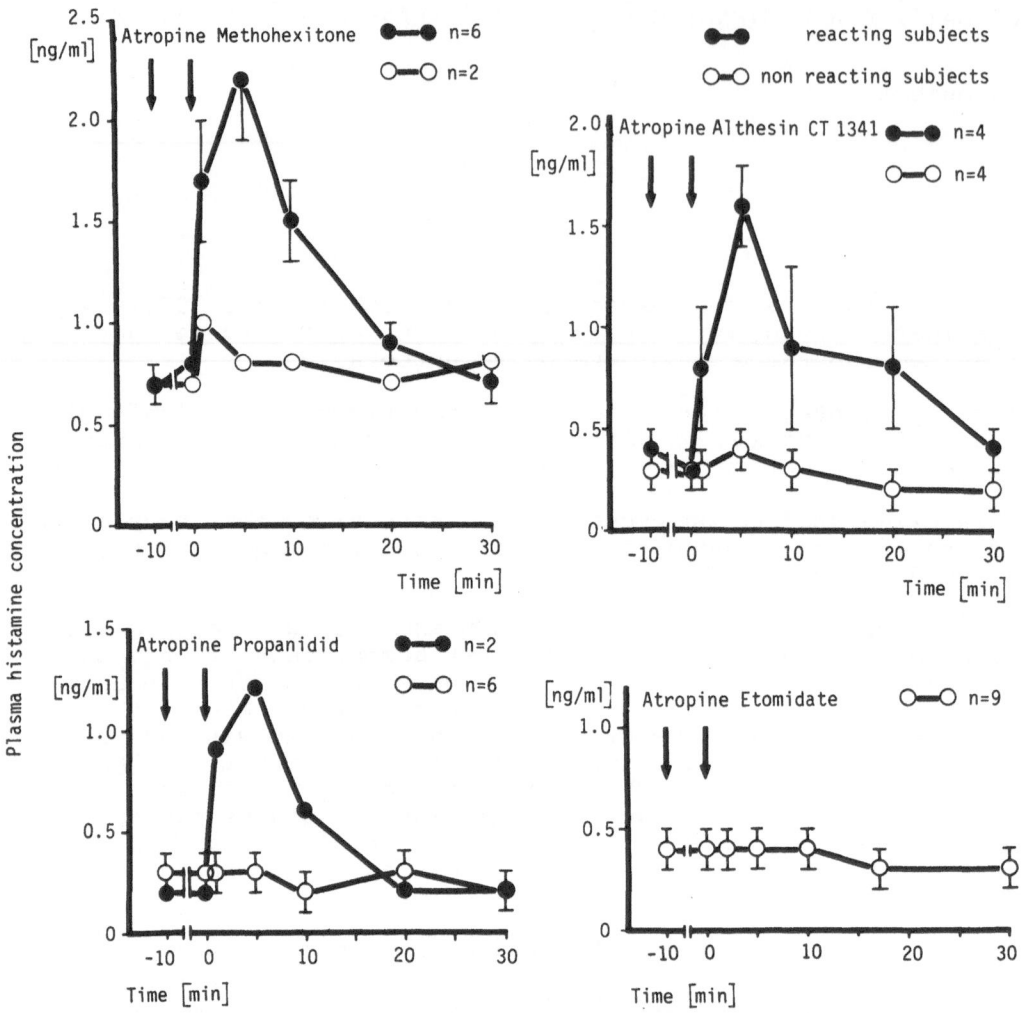

Fig. 1.Histamine release in several test persons following the injection of anaesthetic drugs

A comparison of 106 inductions of hypnosis with propanidid with 80 etomidate inductions, showed that the latter had virtually no effect on the circulation. Propanidid produced a decrease in the systolic blood pressure of about 25 % (Fig. 2) whether using the antihistaminic Tavegil as premedication or not. A slowing down of the injection speed for etomidate from 10 to 60 sec did not result in change in blood pressure (Fig. 3). A statistical analysis of these data showed the differences between etomidate and propanidid to be significant (DOENICKE, 1973).

Together with the investigations bearing on the circulation during induction, the subjective and objective experiences of the patients were noted. The most striking side effects after etomidate were more or less marked myoclonias. By myoclonias we mean

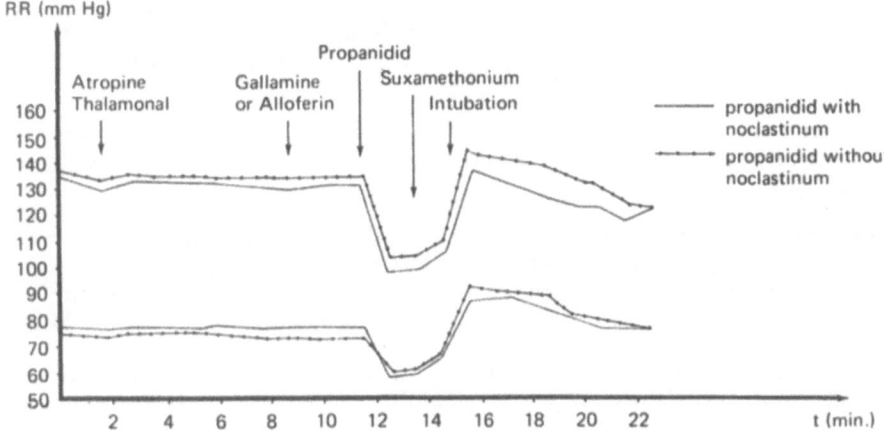

Fig. 2.*Blood pressure during inductionphase with propanidid - 5 mg/kg body-weight - with neclastinum in the premedication (n = 31) as without neclastinum (n = 73)*

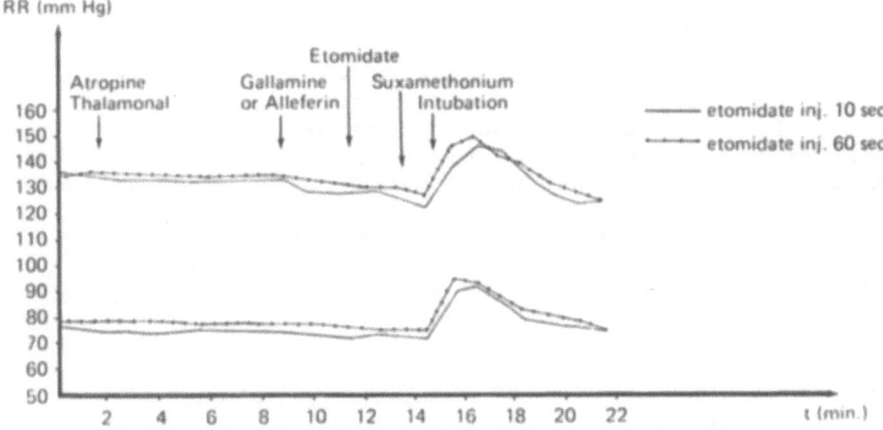

Fig. 3.*Blood pressure during inductionsphase with etomidate - 0.15 mg/kg body-weight - injection speed 10 sec (n = 43) and 60 sec (n = 37)*

uncontrolled and uncoordinated spontaneous movements of either individual or several groups of muscles, particularly affecting the roots of the extremities. We regard them as signs of the release of inhibition or of direct stimulation of the diencephalic/mesencephalic regions. Paroxysmal potentials could never be detected in the EEG.
Several patients suffering from epilepsy were given etomidate with monitoring by EEG and there were no complications.

A double-blind study against propanidid and methohexital was carried out to demonstrate the advantages and disadvantages.
A total of 13 subjects volunteered to undergo treatment at 14-day intervals. After administrating methohexital the blood gas anal-

yses showed significant increase in the PCO_2 and a significant drop in the PO_2. At the stated dosages no changes of any kind in the blood gases could be detected after either propanidid or etomidate.

Blood sugar levels, serum cholinesterase activity and fat metabolism did not significantly change after any of the 3 hypnotics (DOENICKE et al., 1973).

We consider the EEG to be one of the most important parameters for detecting a hypnotic effect. With the doses used in this experiment, the dispersion was large both on propanidid (5 mg/kg b.w.) as well as etomidate (0.15 mg/kg b.w.). Comparing propanidid to methohexital the depth of sleep (1.5 mg/kg b.w.) was significantly increased in the latter, but there was no marked difference between etomidate and methohexital (DOENICKE, 1973; DOENICKE et al., 1973).

The EEG investigations showed that a dose of etomidate (0.15 mg/kg b.w.) corresponds roughly to the hypnotic effect of 6 or 7 mg/kg b.w. of propanidid and 5 mg/kg b.w. of thiopentone. Signs of tiredness after the 10th minute could not be observed after either propanidid or etomidate, but such stages persisted for several hours on experimental subjects after using methohexital and thiopentone.

Our clinical experience and the experimental results have taught us that a dose of 0.15 mg/kg b.w. etomidate often results in a too short and too shallow hypnosis. During operations on out-patients as well as during intubation and transition to inhalation anaesthesia we noticed partly unconscious defence movements.

Further investigations were therefore devoted to determining the safety margin, especially since we knew from the experiments carried out by JANSSEN et al. (1971) on animals that etomidate is particularly superior to the other anaesthetics when safety is concerned.

After the double dose the duration of sleep was prolonged by approx. 2 min. The sleep was considerably deeper and the dispersion in the maximum period of effectiveness was definitely smaller than at a dose of 0.15 mg/kg b.w. Depth and duration of sleep correspond to about those after 1.5 mg methohexital.

The most important aspect for clinical practice, however, is that a second injection produced a marked prolongation of sleep. Myocardial function which was measured during the experiment did not change and there was no stronger depression than the first initial dose (DOENICKE et al., 1974).

The experience in the clinical-pharmacological tests encouraged us to vary application in the patients. For example, we were disturbed by certain side-effects, such as the appearance of myoclonia during and after the injection of etomidate in 30 % of our subjects. This occurred less frequently after stronger premedication, e.g. with Thalamonal or with Diazepam and Fentanyl.

Summary

Etomidate 0.30 mg/kg b.w. is more active than 5 mg/kg b.w. thiopentone or 1.5 mg/kg b.w. methohexitone. At the same time this
dose of etomidate has less side-effects on breathing and
myocardial function. The strong myocardial depression as well as
the drastic changes of blood gases after methohexitone, propanidid
and thiopentone together with a short sleeping period after thiopentone proved that etomidate is a better hypnotic than barbiturates and propanidid.
The interplay of clinical-pharmacological investigations in
volunteers and experience with patients have brought new findings
again and again for the past 30 months. By proceeding slowly,
precisely and continuous consultations with the manufacturers we
are able to accomplish an optimal trial using etomidate nearly in
15.000 narcosis without any complications.

Zusammenfassung

Etomidate in einer Dosierung von 0,3 mg/kg KG ist als Hypnotikum
stärker wirksam als 5 mg/kg KG Thiopental oder 1,5 mg/kg Methohexital. Diese Etomidate-Dosis besitzt weniger Nebenwirkungen im
Hinblick auf Atem- und Myocardfunktion.
Die Depression der Atem- und Myocardfunktion ebenso wie die deut-
lichen Veränderungen der Blutgase nach Methohexital, Propanidid
und Thiopental sowie die kürzere hypnotische Wirkzeit nach Thiopental, haben Etomidate als ein besseres Hypnotikum ausgezeich-
net als Barbiturate und Propanidid.
Die Ergebnisse der klinisch-pharmakologischen Prüfungen an frei-
willigen Versuchspersonen und die Erfahrungen an Patienten haben
uns im Verlauf der vergangenen 30 Monate immer wieder neue
Erkenntnisse gebracht. Gerade das langsame Vorgehen und die lau-
fende Rücksprache mit dem Hersteller, ermöglichen eine optimale
Erprobung ohne Komplikation bei nahezu 15.000 Narkosen mit
Etomidate.

References

1. DOENICKE, A.: Klinisch-experimentelle Untersuchungen und erster klini-
    scher Erfahrungsbericht über ein neues i.v. Hypnotikum. Proceedings:
    6. Internationaler Fortbildungskurs für klinische Anaesthesiologie,
    Wien, 21.-25. Mai 1973.

2. DOENICKE, A., GABANY, D., LEMCKE, H., SCHÜRK-BULICH, M.: Kreislaufver-
    halten nach 3 kurzwirkenden i.v. Hypnotika Etomidate, Propanidid, Metho-
    hexital. Anaesthesist 23, 108 (1974).

3. DOENICKE, A., KUGLER, J.: Etomidate - Erste klinische Prüfung eines neuen
    intravenösen Hypnotikums. Unveröffentlicht, 1972.

4. DOENICKE, A., KUGLER, J., PENZEL, G., LAUB, M., KILLIAN, I., KALMAR, L.,
    BEZECNY, H.: Hirnfunktion und Toleranzbreite nach Etomidate, einem neuen
    barbituratfreien i.v. applizierbaren Hypnotikum. Anaesthesist 22, 357
    (1973).

5. DOENICKE, A., LORENZ, W., BEIGL, R., BEZECNY, H., UHLIG, G., KALMAR, L., PRAETORIUS, B., MANN, G.: Histamine release after intravenous application of short-acting hypnotics. A comparison of Etomidate, Althesin (T 1341) and Propanidid. Brit.J.Anaesth. <u>45</u>, 1097 (1973).

6. DOENICKE, A., WAGNER, E., BEETZ, K.H.: Blutgasanalysen (arteriell) nach drei kurzwirkenden i.v. Hypnotika (Propanidid, Etomidate, Methohexital). Anaesthesist <u>22</u>, 353 (1973).

7. JANSSEN, P.A.J., NIEMEGEERS, C.J.E., SCHELLEKENS, K.H.L., LENAERTS, F.M.: Etomidate, R-(+)-Ethyl-1-(⍺-methylbenzyl) imidazole-5-carboxylate (R 16 659), a potent, short-acting and relatively atoxic intravenous hypnotic agent in rats. Arzneimittel-Forsch. <u>21</u>, 1234 (1971).

8. LORENZ, W., DOENICKE, A., MEYER, R., REIMANN, H.J., KUSCHE, J., BARTH, H., GESING, H., HUTZEL, M., WEISSENBACHER, B.: Histaminerelease in man by Propanidid and Thiopentone: Pharmacological effects and clinical consequences. Brit.J.Anaesth. <u>44</u>, 355 (1972).

The EEG after Etomidate

J. Kugler, A. Doenicke and M. Laub

The Problem

Following the experimental determinations of the hypnotic effect
of etomidate in animals and in clinical experiments carried out
so far, and on the basis of the available anaesthesiological
experience, it seemed justified to test the usefulness of etomidate in combined balanced anaesthesia by further investigations
with electroencephalographic control. In our earlier publication
(DOENICKE et al., 1973) we described the essential similarity
of the course of the EEG stages in etomidate anaesthesias to the
stages in barbiturate anaesthesias and determined the tolerance
of healthy subjects to an etomidate dose of 0.15 mg/kg. These
findings and the observations of other authors now led to ques-
tions, which we tried to clarify by means of a clinical experimental investigation. The aim was to establish whether:

1. etomidate causes - also in the higher doses required for
    anaesthesia in adults - EEG stages which correspond to the
    known stages with other intravenously applied anaesthetics;

2. the combination with a premedication of diazepam and fentanyl
    influences the courses of the EEG and the clinically notice-
    able signs (especially the motor phenomena);

3. the EEG changes together with the clinical symptoms allow
    any conclusions concerning special action mechanisms of
    etomidate; and

4. any special epileptogenic action of etomidate is detectable.

Material and Method

Etomidate anaesthesias were carried out in 87 healthy subjects
aged 21 - 28, divided into 5 groups. The subjects received different premedications in sequences and at times defined previously.
Etomidate was injected i.v. continuously within 60 sec in each
case. 0.5 mg atropine was administered to each subject 15 min
before induction.

In each test the recording of the EEG was started before the first
premedication and was continued until the 60th minute after the
first etomidate injection, and also from the 75th to the 90th
min, and from the 105th to the 120th min. The EEG was taken by
two bipolar longitudinal rows situated paramedially (10/20-system)
in 8 channels.

Group I

a)   Induction: 0.15 mg/kg of etomidate i.v.; n = 17

b)   Induction: 0.3 mg/kg of etomidate i.v.; n = 28

Group II

          0.1 mg/kg of diazepam 5 min before induction

          0.15 mg/kg of etomidate i.v.; n = 8

Group III

          0.1 mg/kg of diazepam 10 min before induction

          0.3 mg/kg of etomidate
      + 0.15 mg   of fentanyl; n = 10

Group IV

          0.1 mg/kg of diazepam 10 min before induction

          0.15 mg/kg of etomidate (1st injection)

          0.15 mg/kg of etomidate (2nd injection 3 min
                      after end of 1st injection); n = 8

Group V

          0.1 mg/kg of diazepam 10 min before induction

          0.3 mg/kg of etomidate
      + 0.1 mg   of fentanyl

          0.3 mg/kg of etomidate after 4 min

          0.3 mg/kg of etomidate after 12 min
      + 0.05 mg   of fentanyl; n = 16

In some of these EEG leads an electronic analysis was carried out
in real time with sequential power spectra (with 20 sec intervals)
from the right precentral and the right occipital region (using
an AEG/Telefunken B10 16 analyzer).

Simultaneously with the EEG, the ECG I, and oculogram (for measuring the rapid and slow eye movements from the two outer corners
of the eye), a pneumotachogram (for measuring the respiratory
rate), and a mechanogram (for measuring motor activity) were recorded each in one recording channel. The carotid pulse and the
heart sounds were recorded simultaneously with a separate recording system.

After the 60th and the 90th minute of recording, the 15 min pauses
were used to record neurological elementary findings, psycho-
experimental test results, and subjective statements on the

general condition (this will be reported elsewhere: DOENICKE, A., KUGLER, J., 1975).

The EEG curves were evaluated visually by a single doctor, who classified the EEG stages in all successive 40-sec epochs with index values (KUGLER, J., 1966) and then illustrated them on a compressed time-scale in "narcograms".

All the measured values could be used for mean value determinations and for statistical calculations. In the calculation of the significance thresholds, the significance level (p = 5 %) and the degree of freedom were taken into account, and the significance was determined by the Student method.

Observations

Principally, the EEG stages after an injection of 0.3 mg/kg of etomidate resemble the classical stages observed with barbiturates and other anaesthetics: The first noticeable EEG changes already occur during an i.v. injection of 60 sec duration, mostly after a latency period of 30 - 40 sec (the latency period being dependent on the injection rate). These changes consist of diffuse and irregular rapid activity comparable to the "induction stage" with barbiturates. As a rule, they last for several seconds (with a fast injection rate only a few seconds). Then, transition to a mixed activity follows with slow 5 - 3 sec waves superimposed by rapid activity and corresponding to the slight anaesthesia stage (Fig. 1). Subsequently, a higher slow activity develops, corresponding to a medium anaesthesia stage, which in general offers hypnotic and analgesic action that can already be utilized for surgical purposes (Fig. 1, right). The slow activity then increases and the superimposed rapid activity becomes lower and lower. This stage corresponds to deep anaesthesia. The so-called "burst suppression" activity may now follow, i.e., groups of irregular slow waves alternating with intervals of very flat waves lasting for several seconds (sometimes with actual "electro-cerebral inactivity"). This state is usually an expression of exceeding the tolerance limit and of an appreciable functional disturbance in synchronizing brainstem regions.

The EEG allows determination of the stages in arbitrarily chosen epochs (for practical reasons we preferred for the visual analysis those of 40 sec duration), which are then entered onto graphs to illustrate the course of the changes with time (Fig. 2). After the injection of etomidate, these "narcograms" show a rapid transition from the conscious stage to the deep anaesthesia stages and subsequently a rapid subsidence of the anaesthesia, and they indicate the post-anaesthetic oscillations of vigilance (Fig. 2). However, selection of 40-sec epochs for the evaluation means that oscillations of shorter duration are lost.

The narcograms of all the subjects can be superimposed to give "mean-value curves"; beside, the mean value for stages of all successive 40-sec epochs their ranges of scatter can thus also be given. These provide an idea of the variability after administration of identical doses at the same injection rates.

34

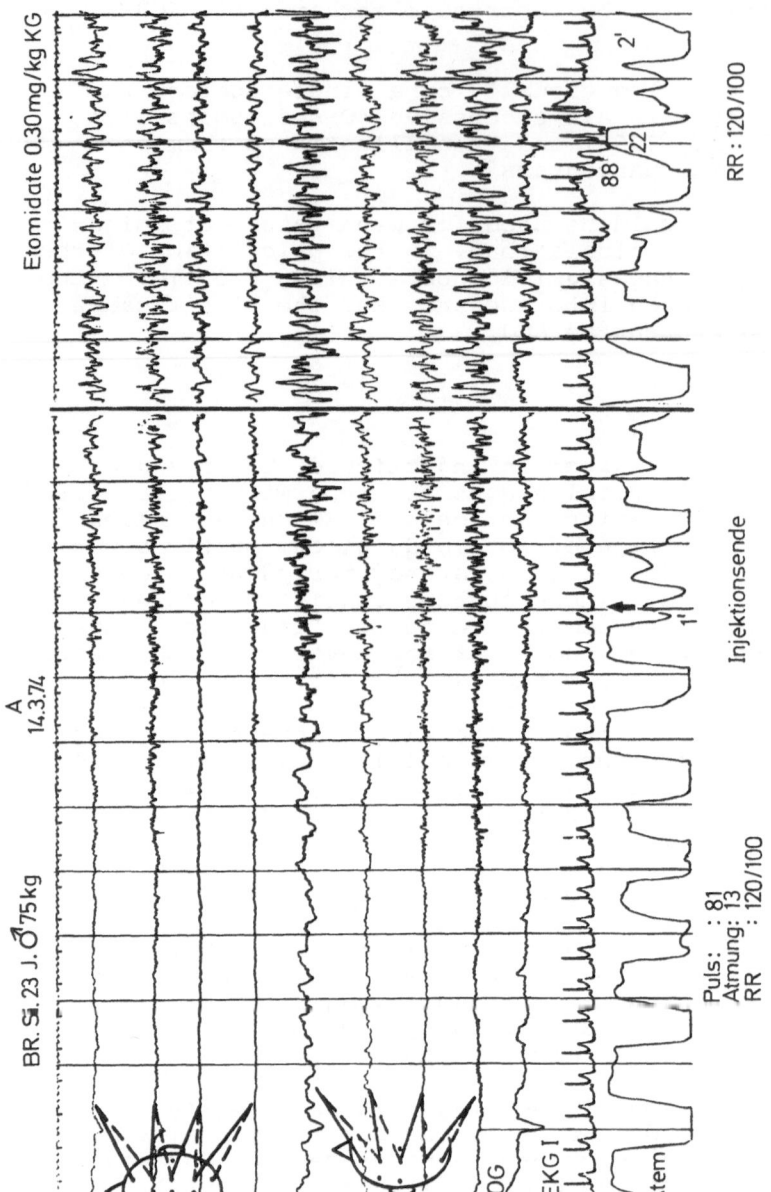

Fig. 1. Etomidate-induced EEG-changes (healthy volunteer): 10 sec before the end of injection (0.3 mg/kg within 1 min) relatively fast irregular activity. At the end of the injection (1', ↑) small slow waves. One minute later (2') high slow activity, superimposed fast waves. The oculogram (OG; right to left epicanthus) shows decreasing rapid eye movements of wakefulness only on the left. In ECG (EKG I) increasing heart rate (up to 88/min.) Respiration (Atem) irregular, relatively fast (22 min)

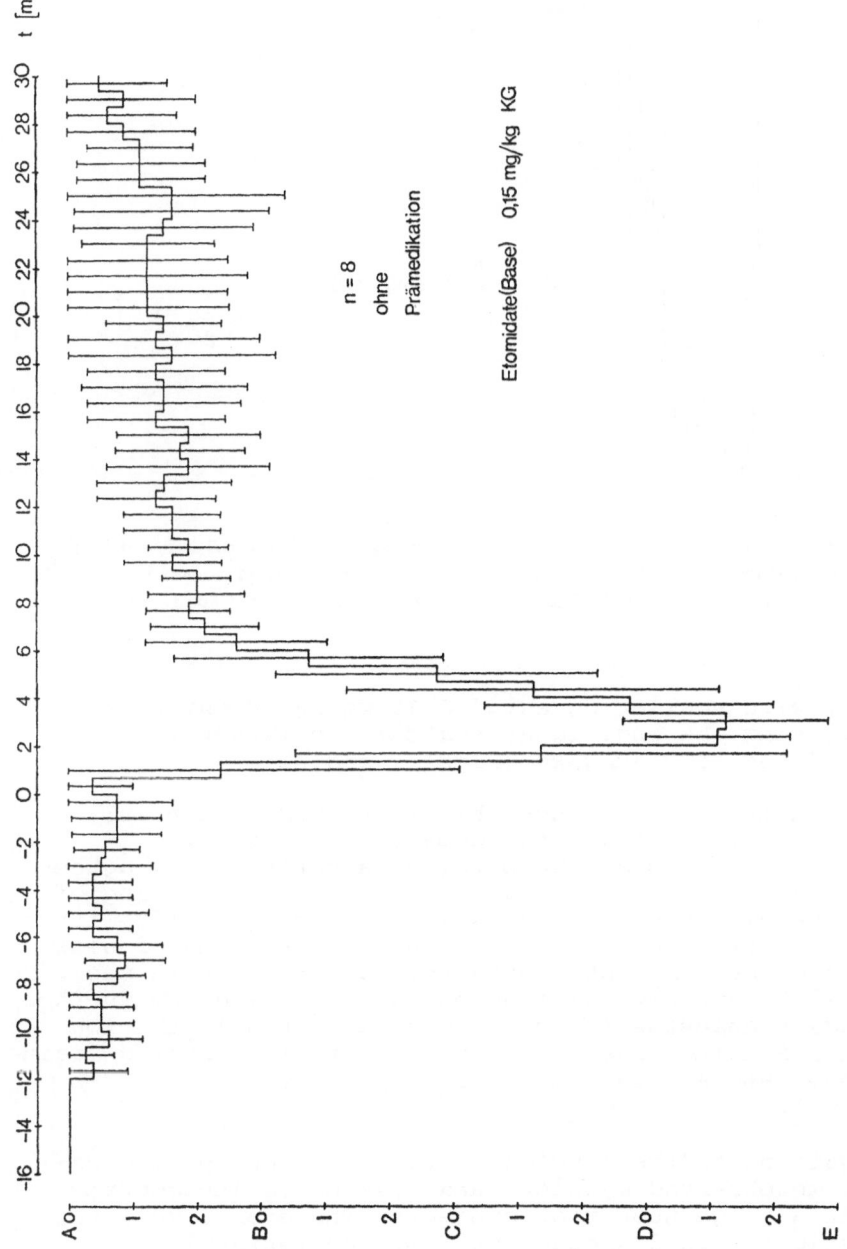

Fig. 2.Narcogram with EEG-stages (A = wakefulness, E = very deep narcotic sleep) of all succeeding 40-sec-epochs in 8 healthy volunteers (mean values and standard deviations). At 0 begin, at 1 end of injection of 0.15 mg/kg etomidate (injection time = 60 sec). Hypnotic state lasting about 5 minutes. States of reduced vigilance lasting for half an hour

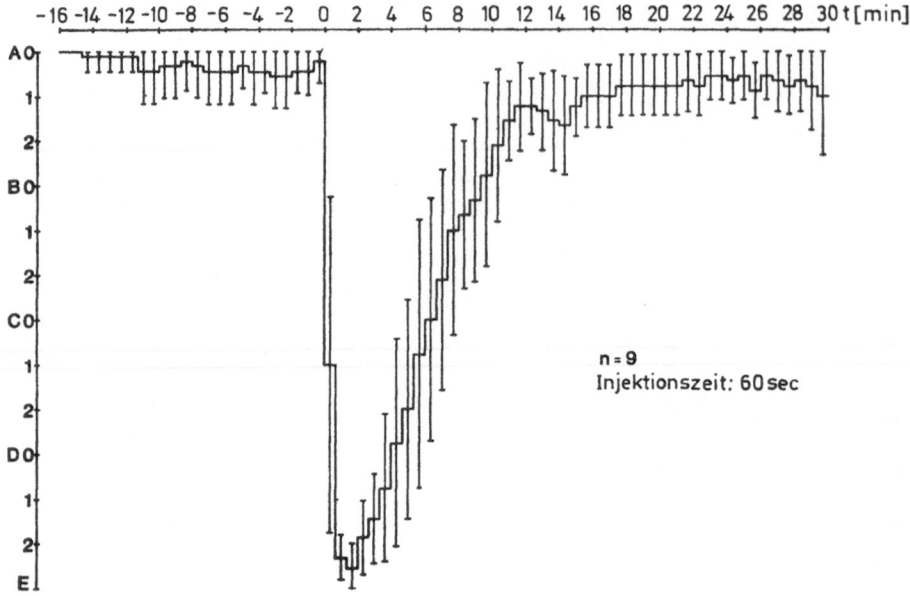

Fig. 3. Narcogram of 9 healthy volunteers. At 0 begin, at 1 end of injection 0.3 mg/kg etomidate. Hypnotic state lasting for about 8 minutes, smaller standard deviations as compared with Fig. 2. States of reduced vigilance 2^h after injection

It is found that with smaller doses of 0.15 mg/kg the standard deviations expressing the individual scatter are larger than with the larger doses of 0.3 mg/kg (Figs. 2 and 3).

With electronic analysers it is possible to record sequential power spectra in "real time" and to compare then with visual evaluations of the EEG records. We obtained a satisfactory agreement with our visual evaluation (Fig. 4). After the beginning of the injection, the electronic analysis showed a rapid shift within the power spectra, with increasing dominance of the band of slow activity and a decrease in alpha activity, particularly in the parieto-occipital leads. Several minutes later, during the further course of etomidate anaesthesia, the power decreased in the low frequency ranges. Simultaneously, irregular activity occured again in the alpha-wave band and the amount of rapid activity increased (Fig. 4).

In the investigations of the etomidate stages without premedication (group I), we observed myocloni and dyskinesia (ephemeral hyperkinesia) in a large number of subjects. Therefore, we investigated combinations with diazepam (Valium) and fentanyl.

After the administration of diazepam, already before the beginning of anaesthesia (group II), the EEG showed a transition from consciousness to states of reduced vigilance and slight ephemeral sleepiness. The EEG pattern corresponded to a slowed and lower background activity with diffuse low rapid activity.

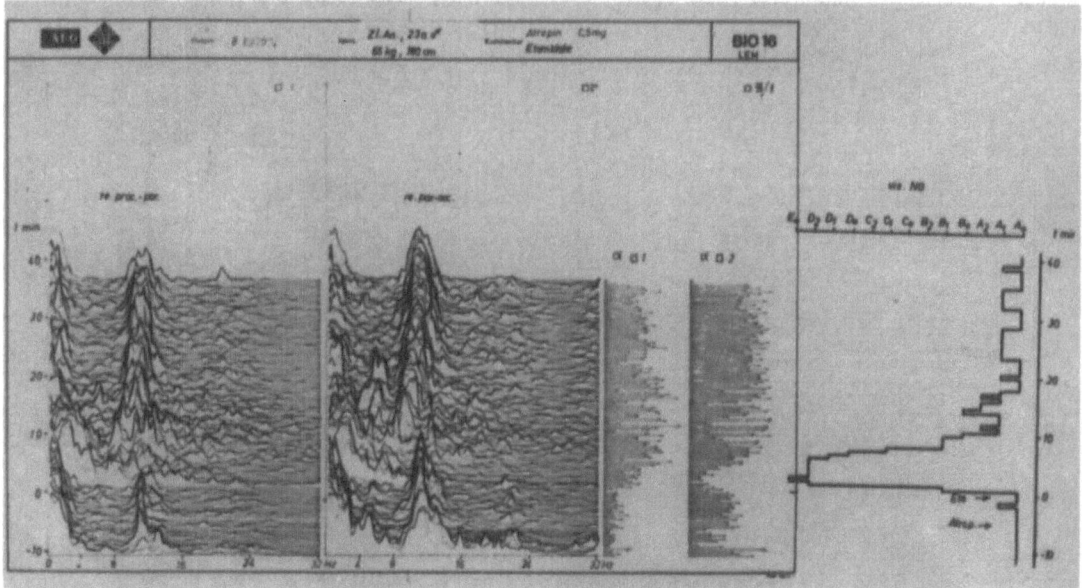

Fig. 4.Sequential power spectra with 20 sec intervals (from bottom to top) right precentral-parietal (re.präc.-par.) and right parieto-occipital (re. par.-occ), intensity of the 8-12/sec frequency range right precentral-parietal (∝□1) and right parieto-occipital (∝□2) and narcogram. Volunteer ZI. An., injection of 0.23 mg/kg etomidate

At the beginning of anaesthesia the initial EEG-activity returned for a short period of time, obviously because the subjects paid attention to the preparations for the intravenous injection (Fig. 5). After the intravenous induction the transition to the medium and deep sleep stages was faster than after the injection of etomidate alone. The narcogram (Fig. 5) also showed a longer duration of the deep and medium anaesthesia stages than without diazepam, and in several subjects oven deeper stages of anaesthesia. The subsidence of the anaesthesia was retarded. Stages of sleepiness or reduced vigilance remained until 30 min. and more after the end of anaesthesia.

Electronic analysis of the combination of etomidate with diazepam (Fig. 6) showed increased irregular rapid activity and appearance of underlying slower waves after the diazepam injection. After the etomidate injection the activity in the slow-frequency range remained longer. After the actual anaesthesia stages (after about the 20th minute) diffuse rapid activity started again, which was absent after etomidate without diazepam (Fig. 4). This was attributed to the longer-lasting action of diazepam (Fig. 6).

The motor phenomena were reduced after etomidate in combination with 10 mg diazepam, but not eliminated. Therefore, we tried the addition of fentanyl (group III). There was also another reason for trying fentanyl: since etomidate lacks a sufficiently analgesic action, it is unsuitable for monoanaesthesia and has to be combined with an analgesic.

38

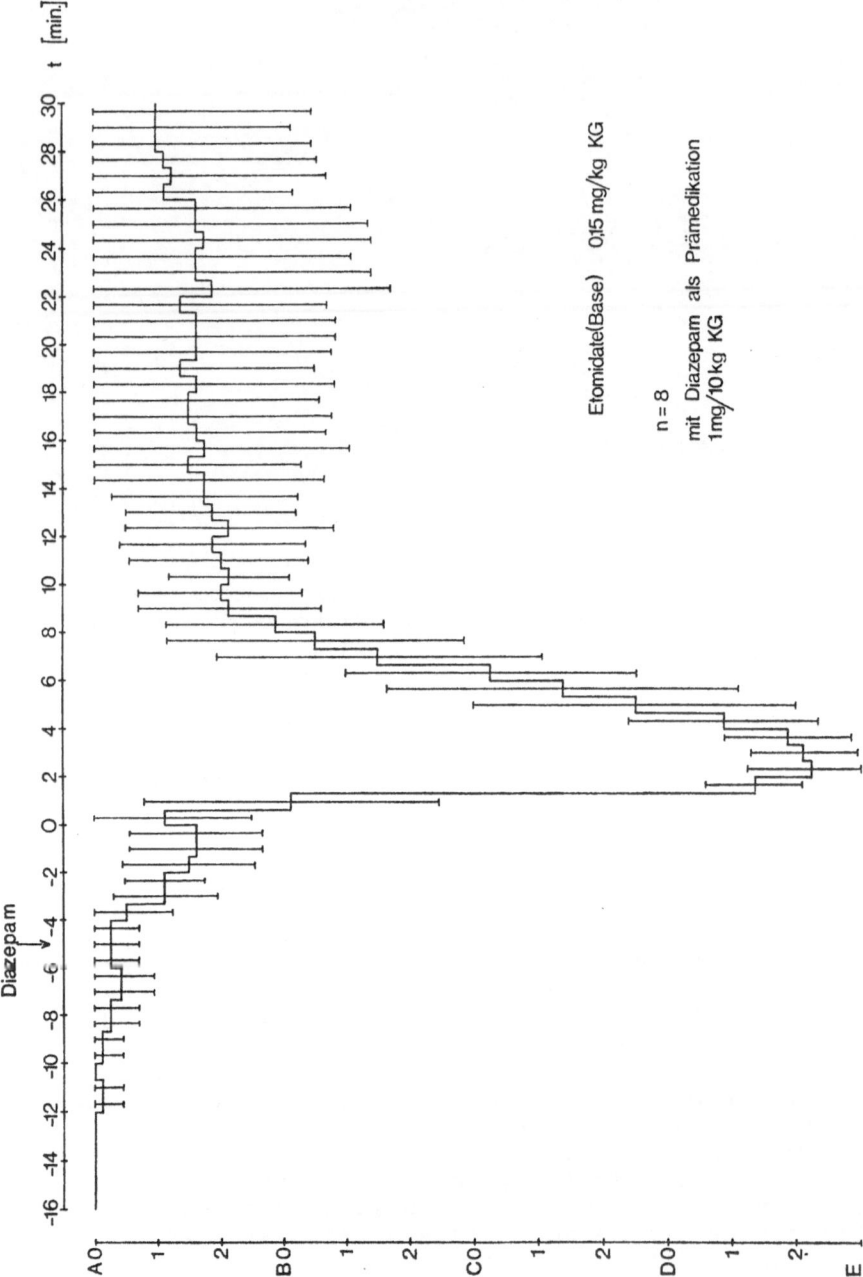

Fig. 5. Narcogram of 8 healthy volunteers. At 0 begin, at 1 end of injection of 0.15 mg/kg etomidate, (injection time = 60 sec), 5 minutes before injection of 1 mg/10 kg diazepam. After diazepam reduced vigilance. After etomidate hypnotic state lasting for about 7 minutes. States of reduced vigilance lasting for more than half an hour

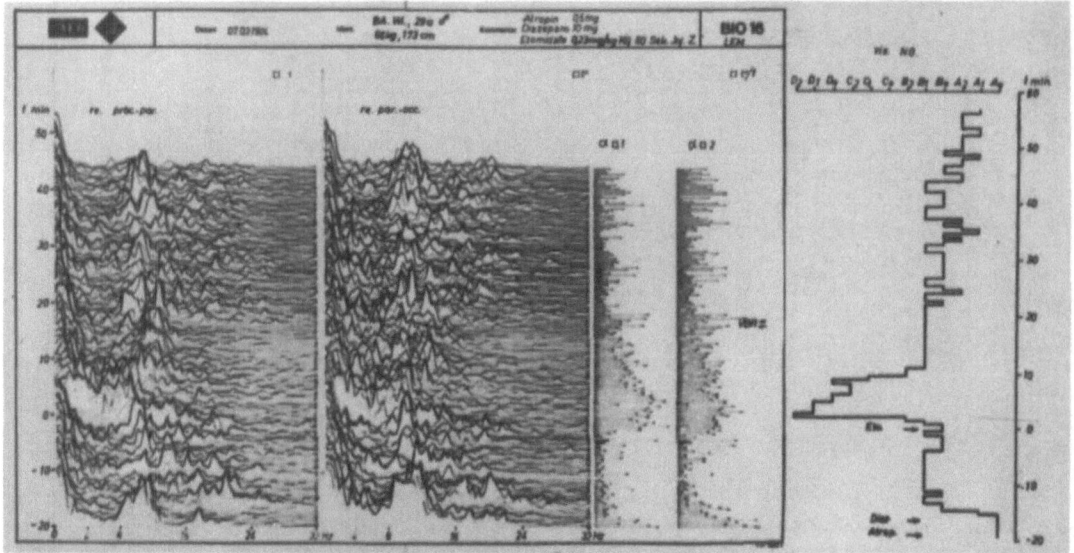

Fig. 6.Sequential power spectra. Injection of 10 mg diazepam. After diazepam activated fast waves, intensity of ⍺-waves diminished, reduced vigilance. After etomidate slow waves longer lasting as in Fig. 4, later on reappearence of fast waves

In the case of the combination of diazepam premedication with intravenous administration of 0.3 mg/kg of etomidate and 0.15 mg of fentanyl the visually determined EEG-stages showed approx. the same course of the medium and deep anaesthesia stages as after the combination of etomidate with diazepam. However, several subjects reached deeper anaesthesia stages than in the previous investigations. The medium anaesthesia stages decreased only after the 8th minute, and slower than after the etomidate-diazepam combination. The stages of slight sleepiness after the 30th min. remained longer; during the follow-up observation for over 2 hours the appearance of vigilance oscillations with ephemeral states of sleepiness was actually noted again (Fig. 7).

The electronic analysis clearly demonstrated these differences. However, the subject in question (Fig. 8) was unusual as far as he exhibited extremely strong activation of the rapid activity after premedication with diazepam and of underlying slow waves over the posterior cranial regions in the initial EEG activity (which was already distinct in Fig. 4). After the anaesthesia a considerable increase in power was noticeable in the lower-frequency ranges, which remained for a longer period of time than after the combination of etomidate with diazepam. Then, an increased proportion of slow waves remained for a long time. It was associated with an increased power in the rapid-frequency ranges, attributable to the addition of diazepam.

After etomidate alone, the slow activity lasted for a shorter time, and even after the combination with diazepam did not remain as long, and is thus probably attributable to the effects of fentanyl (Fig. 8).

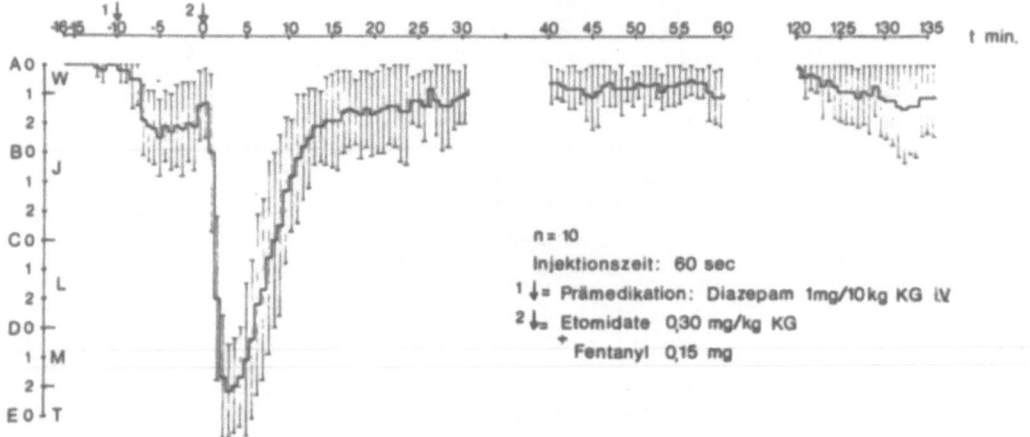

Fig. 7.Narcogram of 10 healthy volunteers. At 0 begin, at 1 end of injection
of 0.3 mg/kg etomidate and 0.15 mg fentanyl. 10 minutes earlier injection of
1 mg/10 kg Diazepam. After Diazepam reduced vigilance (as in Fig. 5). After
etomidate and fentanyl hypnotic state lasting 2 hours after injection (as in
Fig. 3)

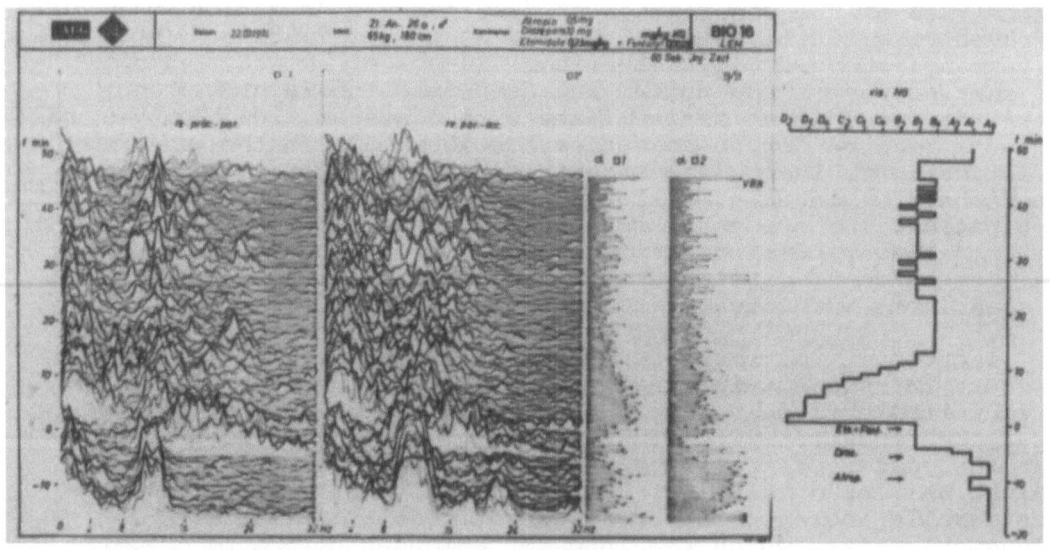

Fig. 8.Sequential power spectra. Same volunteer as in Fig. 4 (ZI. An., 65 kg);
injection of 0.23 mg/kg etomidate and 0.0023 mg/kg fentanyl; 5 min. earlier
injection of 10 mg diazepam. After diazepam activated fast waves, intensity
ofα-waves diminished, reduced vigilance. After etomidate and fentanyl
abundant slow waves longer lasting as in Fig. 6

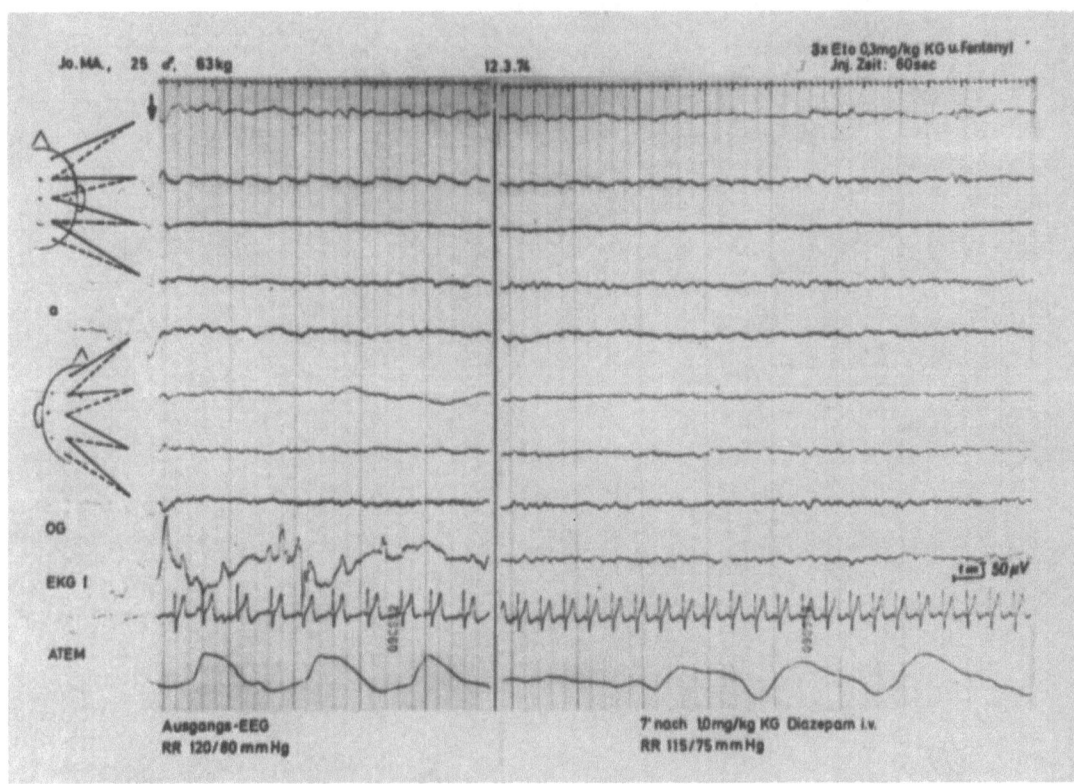

Fig. 9a. Etomidate-induced EEG-changes (healthy volunteer). Part a, left: normal EEG during wakefulness. ∝-rhythm with visual blocking reaction. Okulogram (OG) with rapid eye movements of wakefulness. ECG (EKG) with regular activity. Respiration (Atem) regular. Right: 7^{m} after injection of Diazepam low voltage slow waves and small fast activity, heart rate accelerated, respiration slower

After the combination of etomidate with diazepam and fentanyl, we did not observe any motor side effects in any of the subjects.

In order to test the applicability of etomidate for longer-lasting anaesthesia, we checked the course of the EEG stages after repeated administration of 0.15 mg/kg (group IV) and then after three administrations of 0.3 mg/kg after appropriate premedications (group V). After the first injection the EEG patterns were similar to those after the combination of etomidate with diazepam and fentanyl (Fig. 9a - b). Already after the first injection of 0.3 mg/kg one subject exhibited a transient stage of "burst suppression" activity with series of irregular, slow waves (Fig.9b) and 2-sec intervals with very low activity. On repetition of the injection of 0.3 mg/kg of etomidate 5 min after the first, this stage of "burst suppression" activity was more distinct and lasted longer, for about 1/2 minute: short groups of individual 1-3/sec waves, overlaid by more rapid irregular 4-6/sec waves, lasted for 1-2 sec; the intervals of very low activity lasted for about 3 sec, so that the whole cycle took about 5 sec, which was easily distinguishable from the 3-4 sec respiratory cycles (in the

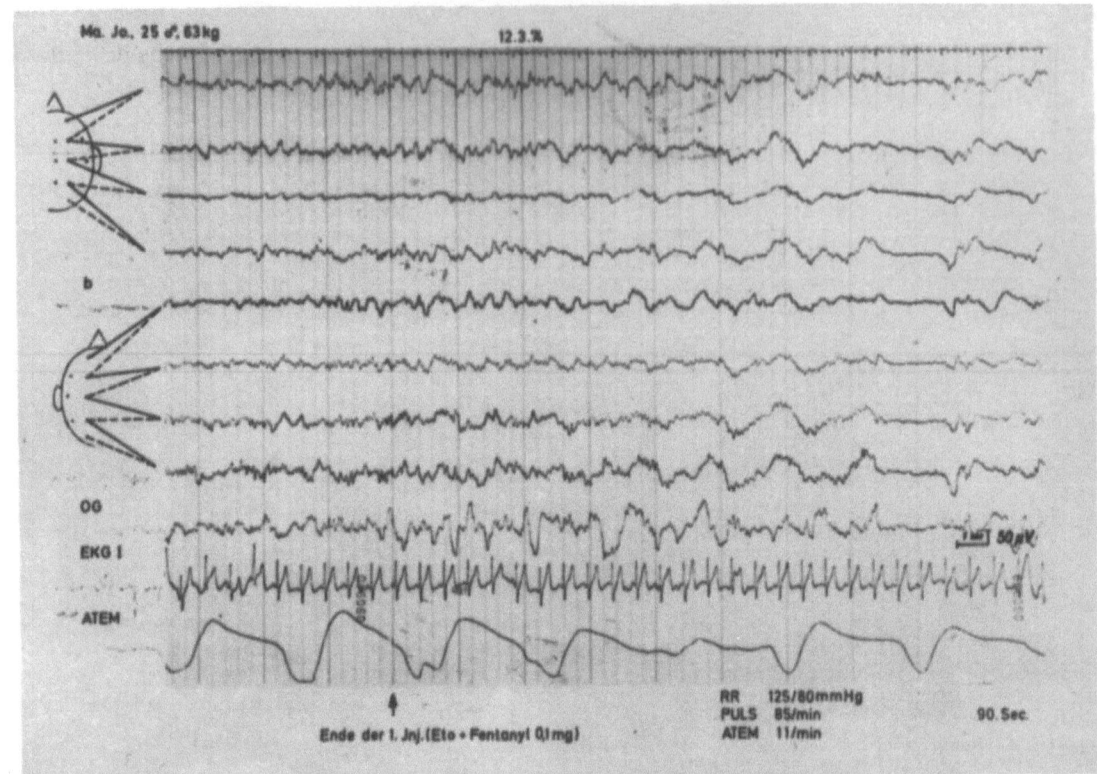

Fig. 9b. Etomidate-induced EEG-changes (healthy volunteer). Part b: 10 sec before the end of 1st injection (↑) of 0.3 mg/kg etomidate and 0.1 mg fentanyl higher irregular fast activity (left) with small slow waves. Within 20 sec increasing slow waves and a first 2-sec-period with very low activity; begin of burst-suppression activity (right)

pneumotachogram, Fig. 9). The "burst suppression" activity expresses the crossing of a tolerance limit and disturbance of the brainstem functions. Its early occurrence in this subject (Fig. 9b) seemed to be based on peculiarities of the individual initial activity, since it started already after the first injection under conditions comparable with those of the combination of etomidate, fentanyl, and diazepam in other subjects (group III). However, the "burst suppression" activity was distinct for a longer time after the second administration (Fig. 9c). It cannot be any peculiarity of etomidate or fentanyl since this form of activity also occurs after barbiturates and many other anaesthetics in correspondingly high doses.

The narcograms for the 8 subjects who received repeated injections clearly showed the changes of the initial EEG-activity caused by diazepam, the rapid onset of anaesthesia after the first injection and the oscillations of the medium and deep anaesthesia stages corresponding to the three injections. After the triple injection the medium anaesthesia stages lasted up to the 20th minute, decreased slowly until the 30th minute, and then slight sleeping stages remained until the 60th minute. Later check-ups, too,

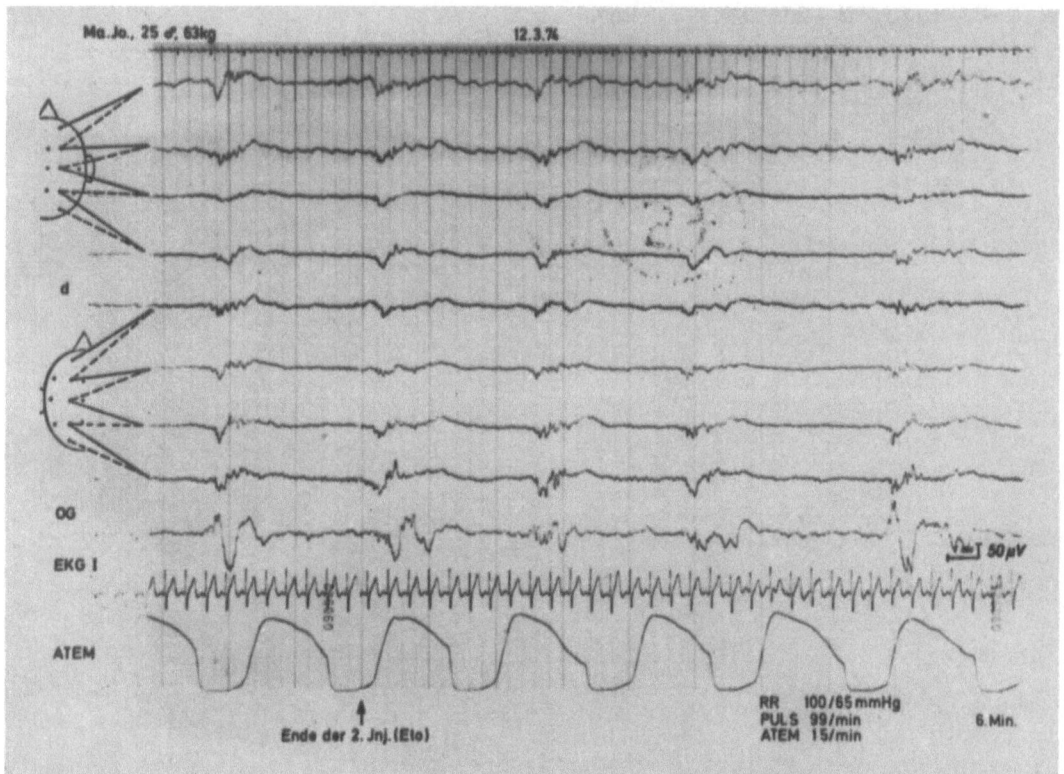

Fig. 9c.Etomidate-induced EEG-changes (healthy volunteer). Part c: burst-suppression activity at the end of 2nd injection (↑) of 0.3 mg/kg etomidate

revealed slight after-sleep stages until the 2nd hour after the injection (Fig. 10). The myocardial function, recorded in parallel, did not show any impairment.

Discussion

The changes provoked in the EEG by etomidate principally correspond to the EEG stages after barbiturates. They depend on the dose, on the injection rate, on the individual initial state and on the combination of etomidate with other agents. In effect, they mean that etomidate exerts a hypnotic effect. They are associated with an impairment of the integrative performance capacity of the neopallium and of the consciousness. In analogy with the experimental findings in animals after barbiturates we can assume that in the induction stage there is a transient activation of cortical neuronal activity. The EEG changes, however, cannot satisfactorily clarify the activity of subcortical structures.

According to anaesthesiological experience, etomidate does not develop sufficient analgesic action. For a reliable assessment of the substance, the EEG observations must therefore be combined with clinical statements.

44

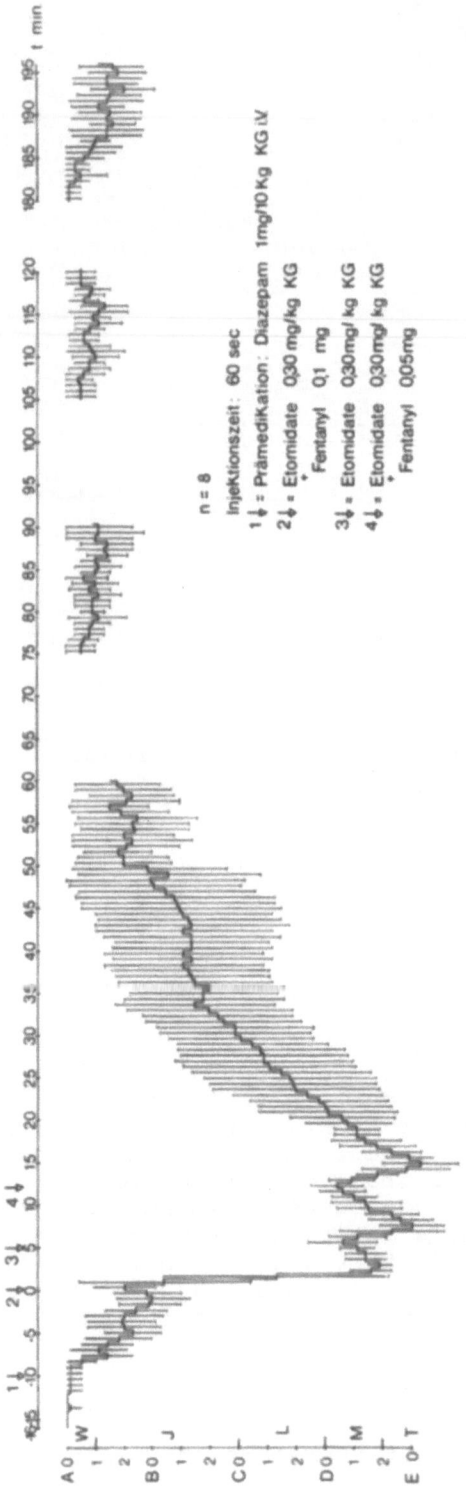

Fig. 10.Narcogram of 8 healthy volunteers. At 0 begin of 1st injection (0.3 mg/kg etomidate and 0.1 mg fentanyl), at 5 begin of 2nd injection (0.3 mg/kg etomidate), at 12 begin of 3rd injection (0.3 mg/kg etomidate and 0.05 mg fentanyl). Hypnotic state lasting for about 25 minutes. States of postnarcotic slight sleep and reduced vigilance lasting for more than 2 hours

The EEG changes and the absence of analgesia and of disorders of respiratory and circulatory functions lead to the assumption that etomidate suppresses cortical functions but does not essentially change the pain conduction in the thalamus or the regulation in the brainstem. The main action of etomidate seems to be exerted on neocortical regions of the telencephalon, whereas the diencephalic, the mesencephalic and the mesencephalic structures are less influenced.

The occurrence of myocloni and dyskinesia (insufficiently coordinated movements) can be explained by a disinhibition of subcortical structures. The regulation of the involuntary and automatic movements lies preferably in the extrapyramidal motor system, which in states of consciousness is subject to the influence of the neopallium. After the transition of induction states into medium and deep anaesthesia the inhibiting cortical influences are usually absent. This assumption is supported by disappearance of the accompanying motor symptoms after the combination of etomidate with diazepam and fentanyl, whose main sites of action lie in the subcortical structures; the influence of diazepam on extrapyramidal motor structures is certain.

Myocloni and dyskinesia (motor automatisms) must not be equated with generalized tonicoclonic epileptic seizures. Myocloni also occur under the physiological conditions of a reduction in cortical activity during physiological sleep as a sign of disinhibition of subcortical structure. So far it has not been possible to observe in the EEG after etomidate definite paroxysmal or recruited epileptic discharges or clinical signs of generalized epileptic seizures. Even in epileptic patients no activation of paroxysms was observed unter etomidate anaesthesia. Thus, etomidate seems to have no convulsant or epileptogenic action.

The suspicion of epileptogenic action in the case of several anaesthetics understandably led to agitation among anaesthetists and to uncritical prejudice, but in general these reports are opposed to experience in anaesthesiological practice: in anaesthesias required for surgical purposes epileptic attacks do occur occasionally, but their incidence is far lower than would be expected from a real convulsant action of the anaesthetics.

Sleep is in general one of the strongest activators of epileptic seizures in everyday life. It develops its triggering action in people with special susceptibility due to genetic or acquired predisposing factors. An EEG check-up in sleep induced by drugs is used in clinical practice for routine examinations where epilepsy is suspected. None of the common sleeping agents have so far exhibited a particular epileptogenic effect. In general, it is the protracted states of sleepiness and falling asleep that give most information in the EEG check-up, while the deep sleep states reduce the electroencephalographic epileptic discharges or eliminate them altogether.

The existing reports on epileptogenic effects of etomidate and other anaesthetics were mostly based on rather unjustifiable conclusions:

1. Motor phenomena were observed in animals and then equated with epileptic seizures in man. Such analogies are, however, unjustified, since the preconditions for epileptic seizures in animals are different from those in man.

2. Occasionally the myoclonic hyperkinetic motor phenomena during anaesthesia were not sufficiently distinguished from generalized tonicoclonic seizures; many a myoclonus or motor automatism may be hidden behind the general statement of paroxysms, which cannot be equated with an epileptic seizure.

Epileptic patients occasionally report attacks "on anaesthesia"; usually, however, the attack only occured at the time of awakening from the anaesthesia, or even on the following morning after a disturbed sleep during the night.

In the past 6 years we ourselves carried out anaesthesia in neuroleptanalgesia with etomidate in three patients with definite generalized primary epilepsy for surgical interventions (after road accidents). In the past 4 years anaesthesias with EEG recording after both propanidid and etomidate induction were carried out in another five epileptic patients. No attack occured during anaesthesia in any of these cases. One patient developed an attack during the post-anaesthetic phase.

3. Many suspicions of epileptogenic action are based on the form of the EEG waves, which have rashly been designated as epileptic discharges, but which do not at all exhibit the required specificity. Apart from this there are authentic reports on paroxysms and epileptic electroencephalographic discharges for nearly all agents used for anaesthesia. (TSCHAKALOW et al., 1975; BUSHART, RITTMEYER, 1965; OROSZ et al., 1972; TOTH et al., 1972; INVERNIZZI, 1964; SZAPPANYOS et al., 1969; GIESE et al., 1974; MICHENFELDER, CUCCHIARA, 1974).

This is opposed to the fact that in clinical and animal experimental comparisons as commonly used for establishing the effects of anti-epileptic agents, an anticonvulsive effect has actually been detected similar to that of diphenylhydantoin, of ketamine (CORSSEN, 1974) and ethrane (BUZELLO et al., 1975).

If steep waves in the EEG are taken for an expression of an epileptogenic effect by some authors it must be replied that steep waves also occur in spontaneous sleep in the form of irregular K complexes as an expression of a working-up of proprioceptive afferences. Their presence after etomidate can be explained by insufficient blockade of afferences from the thalamic structures to the cortex.

Summary

1. The doses of etomidate required for anaesthesia in adults (0.3 mg/kg) lead to EEG changes that are comparable to the classical anaesthesia stages of barbiturates.

2. The combination with diazepam and fentanyl prolongs the stages
of anaesthetic action of etomidate; it suppresses the motor
phenomena (myocloni, dyskinesia) sometimes observed after the
administration of etomidate alone.

3. The EEG changes lead us to assume a hypnotic effect of etomidate which is mainly based on an impairment of neocortical
function. However, etomidate does not produce satisfactory analgesia for surgical interventions, it thus does not seem to
provoke a sufficient blockade of afferences to the thalamic
structures that are important for pain perception. It influences
the centres important for respiratory and circulatory regulation
of the myelencephalon only slightly.

4. We have been unable to detect any specific pharmacodynamic
epileptogenic or convulsant action of etomidate that has been
stated by some authors.

Zusammenfassung

1. Die zu einer Narkose bei erwachsenen Menschen benötigten Dosen
von Etomidate (O,3 mg/kg) führen zu EEG-Veränderungen, die den
klassischen Narkosestadien der Barbiturate vergleichbar sind.

2. Die Kombination mit Diazepam und Fentanyl verlängert die
Stadien der narkotischen Wirkung des Etomidate; sie unterdrückt
die bei alleiniger Gabe von Etomidate bisweilen feststellbaren
motorischen Erscheinungen (Myokloni, Dyskinesien).

3. Die EEG-Veränderungen lassen einen hypnotischen Effekt des
Etomidate annehmen, der hauptsächlich auf einer Beeinträchtigung
der neokortikalen Funktion beruht. Dagegen bewirkt Etomidate
keine für chirurgische Eingriffe befriedigende Analgesie, scheint
somit keine genügende Blockade der Afferenzen zu den für die
Schmerzwahrnehmung wichtigen thalamischen Strukturen zu bewirken.
Es beeinflußt die für Atmungs- und Kreislaufregelung wichtigen
Zentren des Myelenzephalon nur gering.

4. Eine spezifisch-pharmakodynamische epileptogene oder konvulsive
Wirkung des Etomidate, wie sie von einigen Autoren behauptet wird,
konnten wir nicht bestätigen.

References

1. BUSHART, W., RITTMEYER, P.: Befunde bei der Anwendung von Propanidid.
   In: Die intravenöse Kurznarkose mit dem neuen Phenoxyessigsäurederivat
   Propanidid (Epontol). Anaesthesie und Wiederbelebung, Bd. 4. Berlin-
   Heidelberg-New York: Springer 1965.

2. BUZELLO, E., JANTZEN, K., SCHOLLER, K.L.: Der Einfluß von Ethrane auf
   den Elektro- und Pentylentetrazol-Krampf der Maus. Anaesthesist 24, 118
   (1975).

3. CORSSEN, G., LITTLE, S.C.: Ketamin and epilepsy. Anesthesia and Analgesia
   53/2, 319 (1974).

4. DOENICKE, A., KUGLER, J., PENZEL, G., LAUB, M., KALMAR, L., KILLIAN, J., BEZECNY, H.: Hirnfunktion und Toleranzbreite nach Etomidate, einem neuen barbituratfreien i.v. applizierbaren Hypnotikum. Anaesthesist 22, 357 (1973).

5. DOENICKE, A.: Die Beeinflussung der Straßenverkehrsfähigkeit durch die Prämedikation und die verschiedenen Anaesthetika. Zbl. Chir. 101, 230 (1976).

6. GIES, B., GERKING, P., SCHOLLER, K.L.: Das EEG bei Probanden-Narkosen und kontinuierliche EEG-Frequenz-Analyse (EISA) während Operationen unter Ethrane. Anaesthesie und Wiederbelebung, Bd. 84. Berlin-Heidelberg-New York: Springer 1974.

7. INVERNIZZI, G.: Fluothane as an activator in the EEG of children. Electroenceph. Clin. Neurophysiol. 17, 586 (1964).

8. KUGLER, J.: Elektroencephalographie in Klinik und Praxis, 2. Aufl. Stuttgart: Thieme 1966.

9. MICHENFELDER, J.D., CUCCHIARA, R.F.: Canine cerebral oxygen consumption during enflurane anaesthesia and its modification during induced seizures. Anaesthesiology 40, 575 (1974).

10. OROSZ, E., TOTH, S.Z., JUNASZ, J.: Der Einfluß der Neuroleptanalgesie auf die elektrische Aktivität des Gehirns. EEG-EMG 2, 76 (1972).

11. SZAPPANYOS, G., BEAUMANOIR, A., GEMPERLE, G., GEMPERLE, M., MORET, P.: The Effect of Ketamine (Ci-581) on the Cardiovascular and Central Nervous System. Anaesthesiologie und Wiederbelebung, Bd. 40. Berlin-Heidelberg-New York: Springer 1969.

12. TOTH, S.Z., OROSZ, E., JUNASZ, J.: Die Wirkung von Dehydrobenzperidol und Fentanyl auf die cerebrale elektrische Aktivität und Reaktionsfähigkeit der Katze. EEG-EMG 2, 84 (1972).

13. TSCHAKALOW, CH., DRAXLER, V., SPORN, P., SUNDER-PLASSMANN, M.: Zur Wirkung von Propanidid bei Patienten mit erhöhter cerebraler Krampfbereitschaft. Wien.klin.Wschr., April 1975, im Druck.

A Comparison of the Acute Effects of Intravenous Induction Agents (Thiopentone, Methohexitone, Propanidid, Althesin, Ketamine, Piritramide and Etomidate) on Haemodynamics and Myocardial Oxygen Consumption in Dogs

D. Patschke, J.B. Brückner, J.W. Gethmann, J. Tarnow and A. Weymar

Introduction

Daily clinical practice requires an anaesthetic procedure, which helps the patient to fall asleep fast and pleasantly, and which rapidly induces a state of surgical tolerance. Since the pulmonary passage delays an equilibrium between the inspiratory and arterial gas tension of an inhalation anaesthetic and thus extends the onset of anaesthesia (SEVERINGHAUS, 1962), these anaesthetics are not very suitable for the induction. However, the sharp rise of the arterial concentration of an anaesthetic intravenously-administered within a short time has the desired effect. The rapid onset of anaesthesia after the application of a relatively large quantity of an intravenous induction agent is accompanied, however, by uncontrollable side-effects, which might have contributed to the fact, that 10 to 15 % of all deaths observed by GOLDSTEIN and KEATS (1970) during anaesthesia occured during induction. While we now control the depressant effect of injectable anaesthetics upon respiration by artificial ventilation, the circulatory depression is still a considerable risk for the patient. The cardiovascular failure is primarily due to the negative inotropic effect on the myocardium, and/or to the diminution of the venous return caused by peripheral vasodilatation (SOGA, BEER, 1972). The result is a decrease in the systemic blood pressure, and, inspite of a compensatory increase in heart rate, a reduction of cardiac output, which leads to organic hypoperfusion. Although the coronary blood flow is adapted to varying energy demands by intrinsic autoregulatory mechanisms (BRETSCHNEIDER, 1967; GREGG, FISHER, 1963; ROWE, 1974), the acute change of the haemodynamics during induction may produce a negative oxygen balance of the heart, especially in patients, who suffer from circulatory disorders, e.g. hypertension, myocardial and coronary insufficiency, valvular disease, and also shock syndrome. The disturbed cardiac metabolism would increase myocardial depression even more.

Depressant effects on the circulatory system were found with almost all conventional induction agents (VAN ACKERN et al., 1972; BEER and SOGA, 1971; DOENICKE et al., 1974; FISCHER, 1973; SOGA and BEER, 1972; SZAPPANYOS et al., 1969). The only exception seems to be etomidate (R 26 490/ R-(+) ethyl-1 (α-methyl-benzyl) imidazole-5-carboxylate) (BRÜCKNER et al., 1974; DOENICKE et al., 1974; KETTLER et al., 1974; WEYMAR et al., 1974) a potent, short-acting, and relatively atoxic intravenous hypnotic recently developed by Janssen (GODEFROI et al., 1964; JANSSEN et al., morphine-like substances and neurolept-analgesia (GEMPERLE et al., 1966; HEITMANN et al., 1970; KETTLER, 1973; STRAUER, 1972). A comparison of the results of experimental or clinical investigations published so far is only possible within certain limits, however, owing to the difference in the used methods. The present study, therefore, has been designed to compare the acute effects of the barbiturates thiopentone and methohexitone, of propanidid, of the steroid anaesthetic agent Althesin, of ketamine, of etomidate and piritramide on the cardiovascular system under standardized conditions, with particular regard to the coronary blood flow and myocardial oxygen consumption.

Method

The investigations were performed on 48 non-premedicated bastard dogs of both sexes weighing between 25 and 35 kg. After induction of anaesthesia with 3 mg/kg of piritramide (Dipidolor) and orotracheal intubation the animals were normoventilated with a nitrous oxide-oxygen mixture (ratio 2 : 1) – using an Engström respirator with control of the inspiratory O_2 and exspiratory CO_2 concentrations. During preparation of the vessels basic anaesthesia was maintained with small piritramide injections (0.25 mg/kg · h), and a nondepolarizing muscle relaxant was given for muscle relaxation (Alloferin 0.03 mg/kg · h). The acid-base balance was intermittently determined by blood gas analyses, and corrected upon the limits of deviations from the norm. The exposed arteries and veins were cannulated after the administration of 5 mg/kg heparine under radiological control. Every two hours, 2 mg/kg of heparine was administered as a follow-up injection.

Pressure transducers (Statham P 23 Db) were used to measure the blood pressure in the aorta (P_{Aorta}), and the pulmonary trunk ($P_{Art.pulm}$), and also to measure the central venous and left ventricular end-diastolic pressure (P_{LVED}). A catheter tip-manometer (Millar PC 350) facilitated pressure-reading in the left ventricle. The rate of rise in left ventricular pressure (dp/dt) was determined by differentiation (RC coupled) of the pressure curve. The cardiac output (HZV) was determined intermittently by the thermodilution method according to SLAMA-PIIPER (SCHORER, 1967; SLAMA-PIIPER, 1964). The blood flow in the coronary sinus corresponding to 75 % of the blood flow of the left ventricle (HEISS et al., 1973) was measured using BRETSCHNEIDER's pressure difference technique (HENSEL and BRETSCHNEIDER, 1970). The coronary blood flow recorded was related to 100 g of the left ventricle. A CO-oxymeter served to determine the haemoglobine content and oxygen saturation in arterial and coronary venous blood samples (MAAS et al., 1970). From these data the arterio-coronary venous oxygen difference ($AVDO_{2cor}$) was calculated. The total peripheral resistance (W_{ges}) and the coronary vascular resistance (W_{cor}) were calculated from the ratios of the mean aortic pressure minus the central venous pressure (CVP) to the cardiac output and of the mean diastolic pressure minus the CVP to the coronary blood flow per minute and per 100 g of the left ventricle. The product of $AVDO_{2cor}$ and coronary blood flow gave the myocardial oxygen consumption. The heart work was calculated as displacement work ($\bar{P}_{syst}$. HZV/ 100 g left ventricle). In order to calculate the efficiency (η), the heart work was converted into ml O_2/min · 100 g via the caloric energy equivalent (1 mmHg · ml/min = 0.637 10^{-5} ml O_2/min), and related to the myocardial oxygen consumption.

After base-line observations in a circulatory steady-state the following anaesthetics were administered intravenously within 30 seconds.

1.   methohexitone (Brevimytal) in 8 animals at dosages of 2.0 and 4.0 mg/kg

2.   thiopentone (Trapanal) in 6 animals at dosages of 5.0 and 10.0 mg/kg

3.   propanidid (Epontol) in 8 animals at dosages of 5.0 and 10.0 mg/kg

4.   althesin (Glaxo CT 1341) in 8 animals at dosages of 1.0 and 2.0 mg/kg
      For these investigations the animals of the propanidid-group were also used. Since cremophor EL, the solvent of Althesin and propanidid, will release histamine-like substances in dogs (DOENICKE et al., 1973; WIRTH and HOFFMEISTER, 1965), the animals were premedicated 5 hours before beginning the study with an antihistamine, which has proved in a preliminary series to be neutral with respect to the circulation system (Tavegil). Both anaesthetics and doses were injected in a randomized manner. The intervals between repeated doses allowed the controlled parameters to return to the preinjection levels.

5.   etomidate (R 26 490, Janssen) in 13 animals at dosages of 0.4 and 0.8 mg/kg

6.   piritramide (Dipidolor) in 8 animals at dosages of 0.25 and 0.5 mg/kg

7.   ketamine (Ketanest) in 8 animals at dosages of 5.0 and 10.0 mg/kg
      In 3 of these animals the circulatory effect of piritramide had been tested beforehand.

The reaction of the circulatory system was recorded continuously for 20 minutes. At the end of the experiment the animals were killed, the heart was removed, and the left ventricle was weighed. Student's-t-test for matched pairs was used for the statistical evaluation of the circulatory changes.

52

Results

Table 1 shows control values of the measured and calculated haemodynamic parameters under the influence of a piritramide/ nitrous oxide/oxygen basic anaesthesia for each group of experimental animals. The covariance analysis did not show a significant difference between the corresponding control values of the individual animal groups. The circulatory reactions on the higher dosages of the tested induction agents are shown in figs. 1 to 6 in terms of procentual changes against control values. This allows comparisons to be made more easily.

1. Heart-Rate (HF) (Fig. 1)

With the exception of etomidate and piritramide all other induction agents investigated led to a rise in heart rate already 1 minute after intravenous injection.

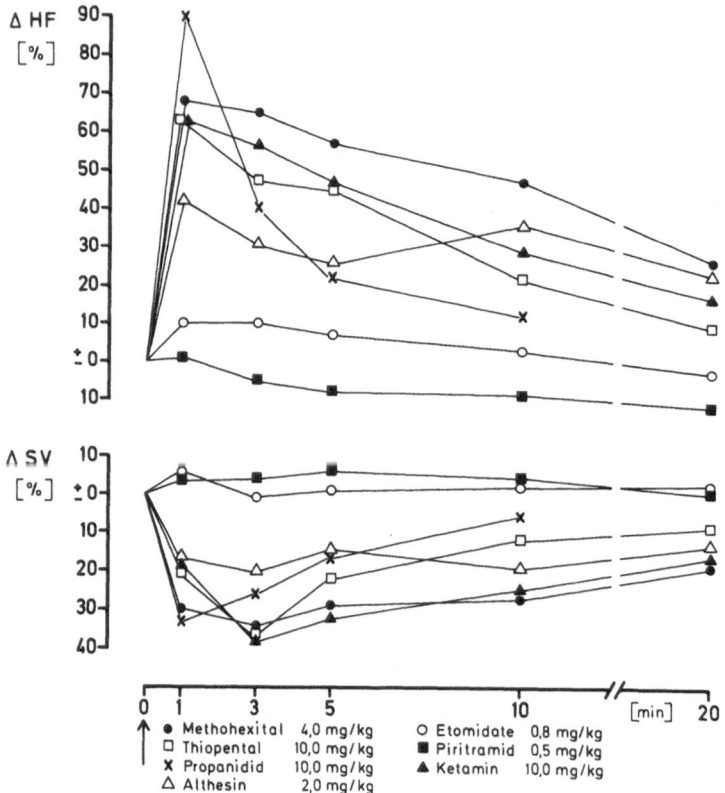

Fig. 1. Change in heart rate (△HF) and stroke volume (△SV) as compared with the control value (△x̄) after the injection of 4,0 mg/kg methohexitone, 10,0 mg/kg thiopentone, 10,0 mg/kg propanidid, 2,0 mg/kg Althesin, 0,8 mg/kg etomidate, 0,5 mg/kg piritramide and 10,0 mg/kg ketamine

This rise was most pronounced after propanidid (90 %), but also conspicuous after methohexitone (68 %), ketamine (63 %), thiopentone (63 %), and Althesin (45 %). While the effect of propanidid on the heart rate had already subsided at the 10th min., the other anaesthetics still showed distinct action at this time (20 - 47 % above control values).

2. Stroke Volume (SV) (Fig. 1)

The reaction of the stroke volumes was almost the opposite of the heart rate. While the maximum decrease after propanidid (33 %) already occured at the 1st min., it was only observed at the 3rd min. after Althesin (20 %), methohexitone (33 %), thiopentone (36 %), and ketamine (37 %). Even after 20 minutes stroke volumes after Althesin, methohexitone, thiopentone, and ketamine were still decreased by 10 -20 %.

3. Cardiac output (HZV), mean arterial pressure ($\overline{P}_{Aorta}$) and peripheral vascular resistance (W_{ges}) (Fig. 2)

Cardiac output, mean arterial pressure and peripheral vascular resistance were only affected essentially at the beginning (1st min). A deviation of the cardiac output exceeding the 10 % range of error of the measuring method was observed after methohexitone (increase by 17 %), Althesin (+ 20 %), propanidid (+ 24 %), ketamine (+ 27 %), and thiopentone (+ 30 %), while the total peripheral resistance decreased by more than 20 % after thiopentone (- 29 %), methohexitone (- 31 %), propanidid (- 35 %), and ketamine (- 40 %). A decrease of the mean arterial pressure by more than 10 % was only observed after propanidid, methohexitone, and ketamine.

4. Left ventricular end-diastolic pressure (P_{LVED}) and pulmonary arterial pressure ($\overline{P}_{Art.pulm}$) (Fig. 3)

The equidirectional changes, though different in extent, of the mean pressure in the pulmonary artery, and of the left ventricular end-diastolic pressure occur within 5 minutes. While the pulmonary arterial pressure only rose distinctly after Althesin (+ 18 %), propanidid (+ 23 %), and thiopentone (+ 40 %), the left ventricular end-diastolic pressure increased by 31 % after ketamine, by 51 % after methohexitone, and even by 80 and 97 % after thiopentone and propanidid respectively. Etomidate and piritramide did not affect these haemodynamic parameters.

5. Coronary blood flow ($\dot{V}_{cor}$) and coronary vascular resistance (W_{cor}) (Fig. 4)

In comparison with the remaining anaesthetics the increase in coronary blood flow after propanidid (114 %) was enormous, although limited to a short period (about 3 minutes); a remarkable increase, however, was also recorded after Althesin (47 %),

Table 1. Control values (mean values and their standard deviation are given; $\bar{x} \pm S_{\bar{x}}$) of the heart rate (HF), stroke volume (SV), cardiac output (HZV), mean arterial pressure ($\bar{P}_{Aorta}$), total peripheral resistance (W_{ges}) maximum rate of rise of left ventrucular pressure (dp/dt_{max}), left ventricular end-diastolic pressure (P_{LVED}), mean pulmonary arterial pressure ($\bar{P}_{AP}$), central venous

	Thiopentone n = 6			Methohexitone n = 8			Propanidid n = 8		
HF (n/min)	70	±	6	70	±	4	86	±	8
SV (ml/kg)	1.18	±	0.2	1.16	±	0.08	0.96	±	0.04
HZV (ml/min · kg)	79.1	±	3.3	81.6	±	5.9	81.1	±	5.7
$\bar{P}$ Aorta (mmHg)	114	±	2	115	±	4	119	±	9
W_{ges} (mmHg/ml/min · kg)	1.38	±	0.04	1.37	±	0.09	1.45	±	0.1
dp/dt_{max} (mmHg/sec)	2408	±	181	2300	±	166	2007	±	127
P_{LVED} (mmHg)	8.8	±	2.0	9.2	±	0.7	9.1	±	1.3
$\bar{P}_{AP}$ (mmHg)	16.8	±	1.4	18.3	±	0.9	18.4	±	1.9
CVP (mmHg)	5.6	±	1.2	5.5	±	0.7	4.5	±	1.2
$\dot{V}_{cor}$ (ml/min·100 g)	81	±	6	78	±	7	83	±	10
W_{cor} (mmHg/ml/min ·100 g)	1.32	±	0.1	1.50	±	0.17	1.48	±	0.26
$AVDO_{2\ cor}$ (Vol %)	13.6	±	1.1	13.7	±	0.8	14.1	±	0.8
$M\dot{V}O_2$ (ml/min · 100 g)	10.7	±	0.8	10.2	±	0.9	11.5	±	1.5
Myocardial efficiency (%)	17.1	±	2.6	17.7	±	1.9	16.4	±	2.6

pressure (CVP), coronary blood flow ($\dot{V}_{cor}$), coronary vascular resistance (W_{cor}), arterio-coronary venous difference in oxygen ($AVDO_{2\ cor}$), myocardial oxygen consumption ($M\dot{V}O_2$), and of the efficiency of cardiac work (η) in each animal group. The induction agents under investigation are: thiopentone, methohexitone, propanidid, althesin, ketamine, piritramide, and etomidate.

Althesin n = 8		Ketamine n = 8		Piritramide n = 8		Etomidate n = 13	
86 ± 7		81 ± 3		77 ± 5		80 ± 6	
1.06 ± 0.03		1.50 ± 0.07		1.36 ± 0.11		1.10 ± 0.08	
91.0 ± 6.1		120 ± 5 4		96.5 ± 4.7		85.2 ± 6	
118 ± 7		125 ± 7		120 ± 9		129 ± 4	
1.25 ± 0.12		1.02 ± 0.05		1.18 ± 0.09		1.51 ± 0.1	
2188 ± 197		2325 ± 168		2338 ± 189		2000 ± 132	
9.6 ± 1.1		9.0 ± 1.3		10.7 ± 1.5		7.8 ± 1.2	
18.2 ± 1.5		17.6 ± 0.8		17.9 ± 1.1		18.6 ± 1.4	
6.3 ± 0.9		3.4 ± 0.8		6.4 ± 1.2		3.3 ± 0.8	
81 ± 8		78 ± 4		85 ± 9		87 ± 7	
1.43 ± 0.2		1.51 ± 0.06		1.40 ± 0.2		1.48 ± 0.15	
14.1 ± 1.0		14.3 ± 0.6		14.4 ± 0.7		14.1 ± 0.8	
11.3 ± 1.2		11.1 ± 0.6		12.2 ± 1.3		12.0 ± 0.9	
20.0 ± 3.6		21.6 ± 0.8		18.8 ± 2.7		14.5 ± 1.2	

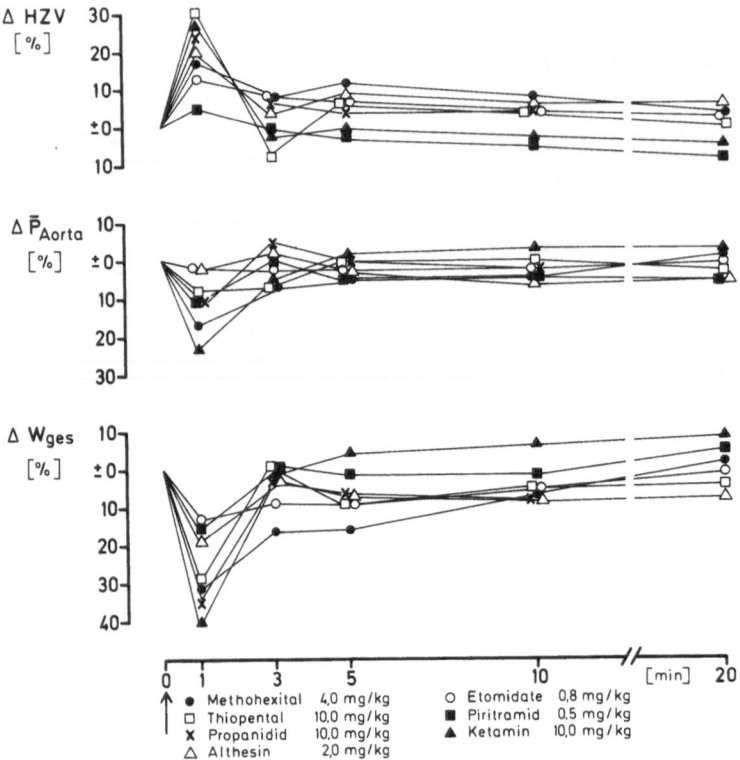

Fig. 2. *Change in cardiac output* (Δ *HZV*), *mean arterial pressure* ($\Delta \bar{P}_{Aorta}$), *and total peripheral resistance* (ΔW_{ges}) *after compound administration (see text fig. 1)*

thiopentone (39 %), methohexitone (38 %), and ketamine (25 %). At the 10th min. after injection of Althesin, thiopentone, and methohexitone coronary perfusion was still more than 15 % above control values, while in the case of propanidid and ketamine these values were reached after 10 and 3 minutes respectively. There were no significant changes after piritramide and etomidate. With the exception of etomidate the coronary vascular resistance decreased by more than 20 % after the administration of all other anaesthetics, the sharpest decrease being 64 % after propanidid. While initial values were reached again within 10 minutes after propanidid, piritramide, and ketamine, the coronary resistance was still 15 % below control values at this time after Althesin, thiopentone, and methohexitone.

6. *Arterio-coronary venous difference (AVDO$_{2cor}$) and myocardial oxygen consumption (MVO$_2$) (Fig. 5)*

While the oxygen difference between arteries and coronary veins remained unaffected under etomidate, it rose by 10 % after methohexitone, by 12 % after thiopentone, and by even 20 % after ketamine within 3 minutes. After 20 minutes thiopentone and ketamine

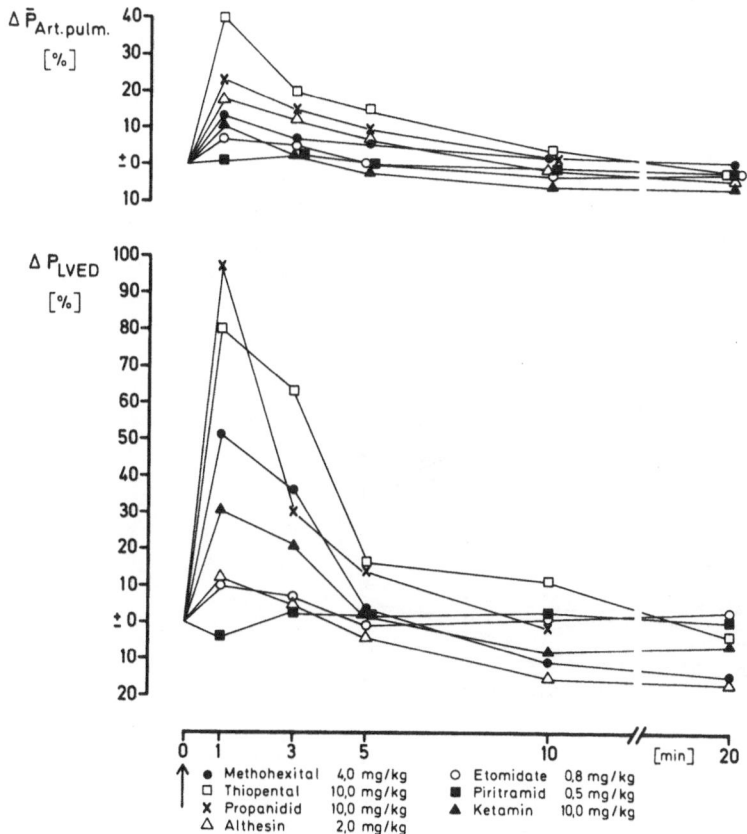

Fig. 3.*Change in mean pulmonary arterial pressure* ($\Delta \bar{P}_{Art.pulm.}$) *and left ventricular end-diastolic pressure* (ΔP_{LVED}) *after compound administration (see text fig. 1)*

values were still 10 % above baseline values. On the other hand there was an initial fall in oxygen content difference after piritramide (- 6 %), Althesin (- 8 %), and after propanidid (- 31 %). Myocardial oxygen consumption remained unaffected after etomidate and even fell after piritramide (- 7 %). The other anaesthetics, however, induced an increase by more than 35 %. At the 10th min. myocardial oxygen consumption still exceeded initial values by 34 % in the case of thiopentone, and by about 20 % in the case of methohexitone and ketamine.

7. *Efficiency of cardiac work* (η) *(Fig. 6)*

The efficiency of cardiac work decreased immediately after the injection of Althesin, thiopentone and propanidid by about 20 %, and by more than 30 % after ketamine and methohexitone. With the exception of propanidid the efficiency remained at 15 % below control values up to the 10th min.

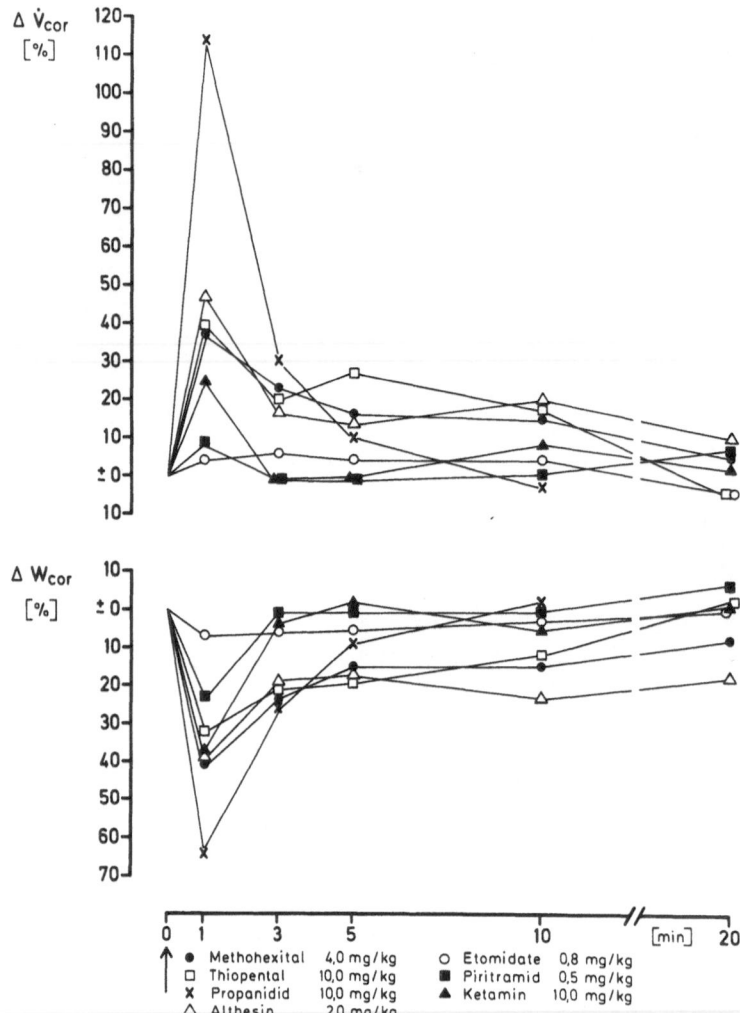

Fig. 4. *Change in coronary blood flow ($\Delta \dot{V}_{cor}$) and coronary vascular resistance (ΔW_{cor}) after the injection of the induction agents under investigation (see text fig. 1)*

8. Inotropism (dp/dt max) (Fig. 6)

While no significant decrease in the maximum rate of rise of left ventricular pressure was observed after etomidate and piritramide, the inotropic parameter dp/dt max fell by more than 40 % immediately after injecting methohexitone and ketamine, by about 30 % after Althesin and thiopentone, and by 20 % after propanidid. Except for propanidid the effect had not fully subsided after 20 minutes.

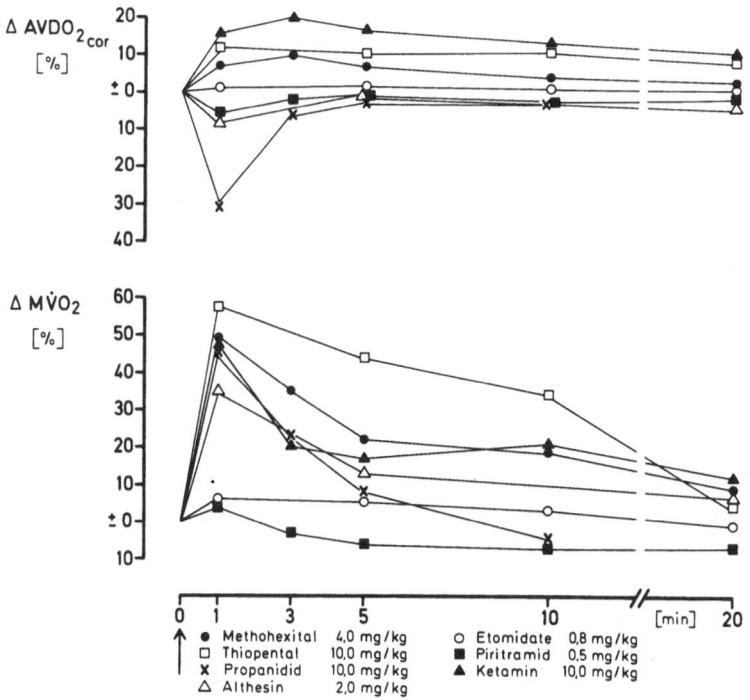

Fig. 5. *Change of the arterio-coronary venous oxygen difference ($\Delta AVDO_{2 \ cor}$) and myocardial oxygen consumption ($\Delta M\dot{V}O_2$) after compound administration (see text fig. 1)*

Fig. 7 to 9 show the maximum changes of recorded or calculated haemodynamic parameters after administration of the smaller dosages of the tested induction agents in the form of column diagrams. As compared with higher dosages the circulatory reaction observed were of a similar quality, but less pronounced.

Discussion

The different methods of clinical and experimental investigations concerning the circulatory effects of intravenous induction agents do not permit a direct comparison of the results published so far. We, therefore, conducted our experiments under standardized conditions in order to obtain the same baseline conditions for each animal group. The electrolyte- and acid-base status was balanced, and possible secondary effects on the cardiovascular system on account of the depressant effect of the investigated anaesthetics upon respiration were avoided by normoventilation. We used piritramide for the necessary basic anaesthesia, since this drug has been proven not to affect the circulation, as was the unanimous result of several investigations (HEITMANN et al., 1970; HEMPELMANN et al., 1971; KETTLER et al., 1971), and apparently,

60

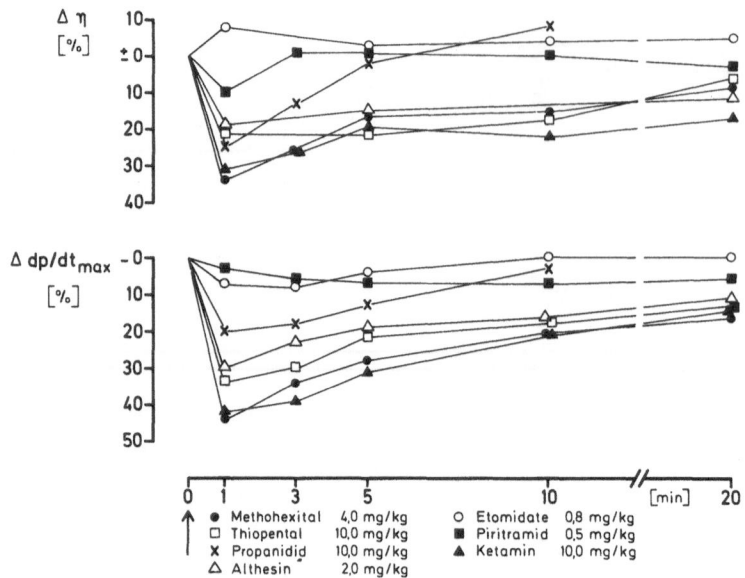

Fig. 6. *Change in efficiency of cardiac work* $(\Delta \eta)$ *and inotropic parameter*
dp/dt_{max} $(\Delta dp/dt_{max})$ *(see text fig. 1)*

does not cause a myocardial depression in contrast to other
anaesthetics as for example halothane. This statement is corrob-
orated by the fact, that the measured control values largely
agree with the haemodynamic parameters of the conscious dog
(O'ROURKE, BISHOP, 1971).

Nevertheless a comparison of the circulatory reactions even under
the above mentioned conditions, and a utilization of the experimental results for clinical purposes is only possible with certain reservations.

1. An interference of the basic anaesthetic with the anaesthetics under investigation cannot be excluded. We did not
   observe, for instance, the rise in blood pressure, and total
   peripheral resistance typical of the conscious subject after
   ketamine (HENSEL et al., 1972; LUTZ et al., 1972, TRABER
   et al., 1970), but even recorded a decrease. This finding
   is confirmed by several investigators (VAN ACKERN et al.,
   1972; FISCHER, 1973; HENSEL et al., 1972). The cocaine-like
   effect of ketamine apparently does not appear under the
   influence of a basic anaesthesia (MONTEL et al., 1973;
   MUSCHOLL, 1973; SZAPPANYOS et al., 1969).

2. A quantitative comparison of the cardiovascular effects
   implies equianaesthetic dosages. While in the case of inhalation anaesthetics the definition of equipotency seems to
   have been carried out in a satisfactory manner by determining the minimum alveolar and end-expiratory anaesthetic

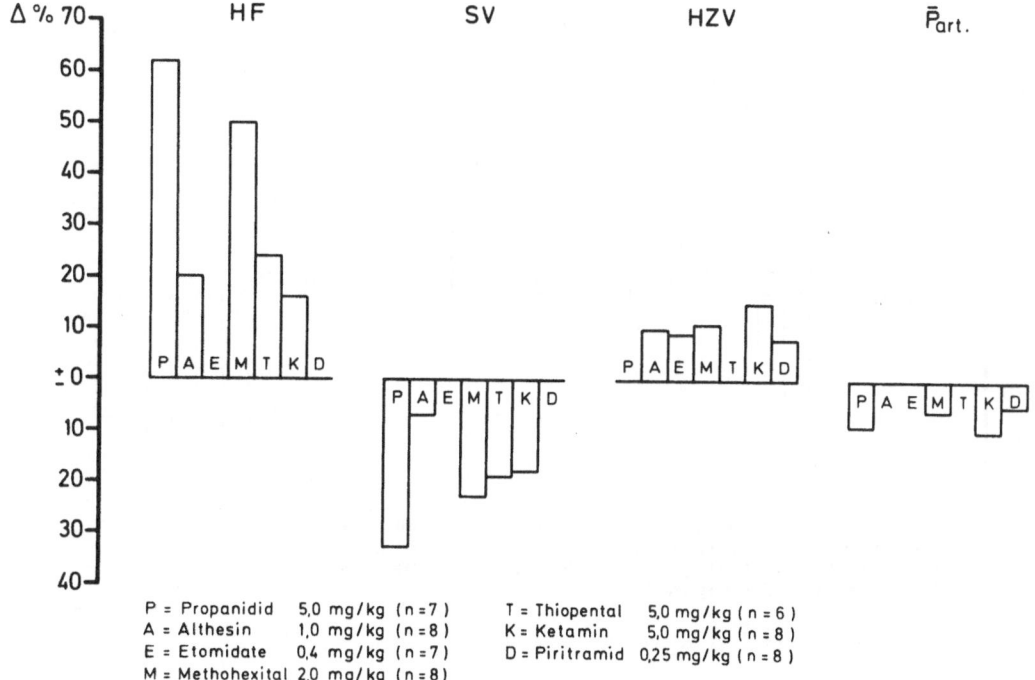

Fig. 7. *Effect of 5.0 mg/kg propanidid (P), 1.0 mg/kg althesin (A), 0.4 mg/kg etomidate (E), 2.0 mg/kg methohexitone (M), 5.0 mg/kg thiopentone (T), 5.0 mg/kg ketamine (K), and 0.25 mg/kg piritramide (D) on heart rate, stroke volume, cardiac output and mean arterial pressure. As compared with the control values the maximum changes ($\bar{x}_{max}$) are given*

concentration (MAC) respectively, where 50 % of all animals tolerate a defined pain stimulus (EGER et al., 1965), no convincing method of determining equipotent dosages of different intravenous anaesthetics has been developed so far.

3. Although according to the unanimous opinion of LOCHNER (1971), GREGG and FISHER (1963) and ROWE (1974) there is no species specific difference between the circulation of dog and man – especially in respect of the coronary circulation – we cannot exclude the fact, that the reactions on the anaesthetic dosage applied may vary from species to species. In veterinary medicine for instance, anaesthesia in dogs is induced with twice to four times the dosage that is used in man (SOGA and BEER, 1972).

Since the haemodynamic responses to the smaller doses differed only quantitatively from those to the larger doses, we restrict our discussion upon the latter. Our cardiovascular studies in dogs showed despite of a considerable decrease in stroke volume an initial increase in cardiac output after thiopentone, methohexitone, propanidid, Althesin, and ketamine owing to a

62

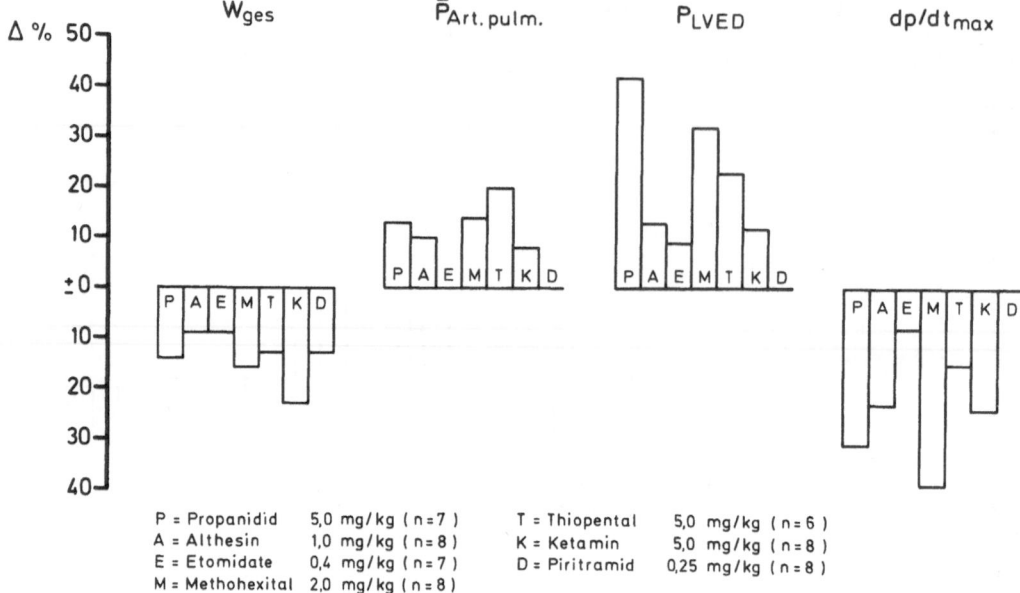

Fig. 8.*Maximum change in total peripheral resistance, mean pulmonary arterial pressure, left ventricular end-diastolic pressure, and maximum dp/dt after compound administration (see text fig. 7)*

simultaneous tachycardia. Besides the barbiturates and ketamine, propanidid had the highest rise in heart rate (more than 60 %).

Since the peripheral total resistance and the cardiac output reacted reversely to each other, the mean arterial pressure remained largely unaffected. The blood pressure only decreased by more than 15 % after methohexitone and ketamine, since the increase in cardiac output apparently could not fully compensate the more pronounced reduction in the total peripheral resistance (approx. 30 to 40 %). In this case the decrease in blood pressure has to be attributed to an additive effect of reduced vascular resistance and an additional myocardial depression, the latter being observed after all the above mentioned induction agents. Although the inotropic parameter dp/dt max is not a sufficient measure for the interpretation of myocardial contractility (MASON, 1969; SIEGEL et al., 1964), the reaction of dp/dt max under consideration of heart rate, preload (end-diastolic left ventricular pressure) and afterload (diastolic aortic pressure) suggest a negative inotropic effect of the anaesthetics. Since the rise in preload and heart rate leads to an increase of dp/dt max without a true increase in myocardial contractility (WALLACE et al., 1963), the decrease of cardiac inotropism should probably be rated higher than the figures of the observed decrease of dp/dt max lead to suppose. The minor afterload changes in our experiments probably had only little influence on dp/dt max.

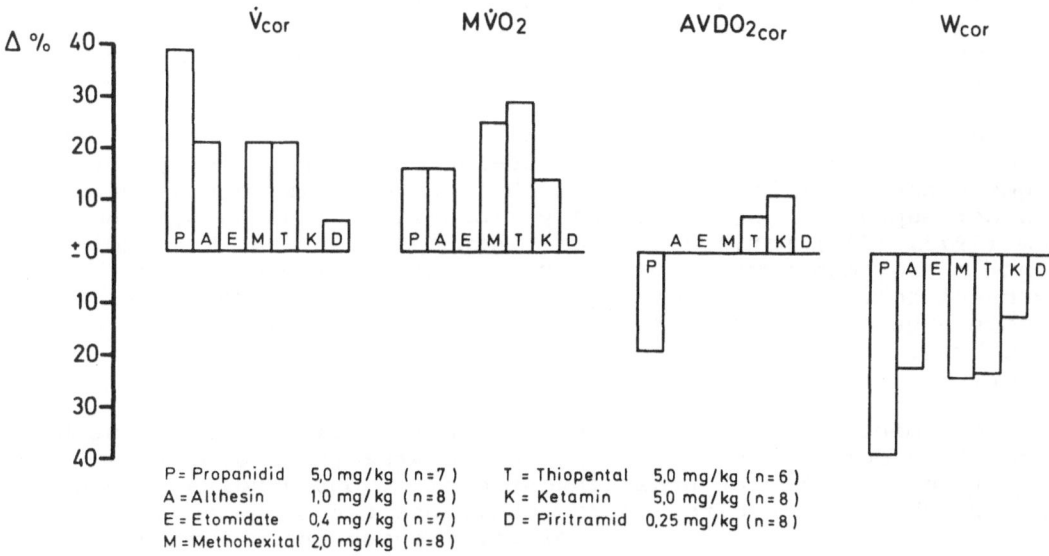

Fig. 9.Maximum change in coronary blood flow, myocardial oxygen consumption, arterio-coronary venous oxygen difference,and coronary vascular resistance after the injection of the smaller doses of the induction agents investigated (see text fig. 7)

Since the reaction of the left ventricular end-diastolic pressure was paralleled with the pulmonary arterial pressure, the rise of the pressure in the pulmonary trunc is believed to be due to the retrograde effect of the increased end-diastolic pressure in the left ventricle, and not to the increased cardiac output or an increased pulmonary vascular resistance. The unchanged central venous pressure in all animal groups after the individual compound administration indicated that the circulatory effects were unlikely accompanied or even caused by diminished venous return resulting from peripheral vasodilatation. The increase in heart rate is probably attributable to a response of the baroreceptors, which have been activated by an imminent hypotension. The induction agents do not seem to possess direct positive chronotropic properties (FISCHER, 1973). Of the anaesthetics under investigation only etomidate and piritramide did not influence haemodynamics and cardiac inotropism, as has been confirmed by other authors (BRÜCKNER et al., 1974; KETTLER, 1973; KETTLER et al., 1974). The unimportant decrease in blood pressure after piritramide is exclusively due to a reduction in total peripheral resistance and not to myocardial depression.

Heart rate, systolic blood pressure, and myocardial contractility are some of the decisive determinants of myocardial energy requirement, while the external cardiac work ($\overline{P}_{syst}$ · cardiac output/kg), and basal metabolism are of minor importance (BRETSCHNEIDER et al., 1970; BRETSCHNEIDER, 1971).

Since a change in the haemodynamics requires an acute adaptation of myocardial energy metabolism, a change in myocardial oxygen consumption after methohexitone, thiopentone, propanidid, Althesin and ketamine may be supposed.

In animal experiments EBERLEIN (1966) as well as KETTLER and his colleagues (1973) could, indeed, observe an increase in myocardial oxygen consumption by up to twice the control value accompanied by a correspnding rise in coronary blood flow, and the SONNTAG team (1973, 1974) noticed the same phenomenon in man. The additional energy consumption is apparently at the expense of an increased heart rate, since cardiac inotropism and myocardial wall tension even decreased. After etomidate and piritramide, on the other hand, no increased myocardial oxygen consumption was observed.

The above mentioned authors effected their studies under constant circulatory conditions in an anaesthetic steady-state of the respective anaesthetics under investigation. Our studies showed, however, that stable circulatory conditions cannot be achieved after customary bolar injection of intravenous induction agents, and that maximum haemodynamic alterations occur within the first three minutes. Using continuous measuring techniques apart from etomidate and piritramide the remaining anaesthetics were found to cause in an anaesthetic unsteady state during induction an initial increase in myocardial oxygen consumption. The adequate supply of oxygen to the heart muscle is guaranteed primarily by the regulation of the coronary blood flow and less by utilization of oxygen. In our experiments the additional oxygen demand, however, was covered in different ways. After Althesin (+ 47 %) and especially after propanidid (+ 114 %) the coronary blood flow increased exceedingly the metabolic requirements, since the arterio-coronary venous oxygen difference decreased significantly at the same time. This observation suggests, that Althesin and propanidid cause a short-term coronary dilatation. Similar properties also have to be attributed to piritramide. Coronary dilatory properties of propanidid have already been previously suggested. DUDZIAK et al (1974), who infused a propanidid-solution into the coronary arteries, discussed a direct action on the coronary blood vessel as well as a diminution of the blood viscosity due to the solvent cremophor EL. The latter point we would like to exclude from discussion, since in a preliminary study cremophor EL turned out to have no effect upon the coronary system. This finding underlines the fact, that the cardiovascular effects after propanidid were not mediated via the release of histamine (WIRTH, HOFFMEISTER, 1975). Although SMITH et al (1973) found even a decrease in myocardial oxygen consumption, the authors observed an initial rise in coronary blood flow - so did BETANCOURT (1970) - and in oxygen saturation of the coronary venous blood. The conflicting data concerning the myocardial energy demand are probably attributed to the unphysiological haemodynamic state of the experimental animals used. After the application of barbiturates, however, and especially after ketamine, additional myocardial oxygen consumption was met by increased coronary flow, and increased oxygen utilization manifesting itself in a significant decrease of oxygen saturation of the coronary venous blood or in an increased arterio-coronary venous oxygen difference.

This finding has to be interpreted in the light of a primary coronary-constrictive effect of the barbiturates and ketamine, superimposed by a secondary coronary dilatation of metabolic origin[1].

The cardiac efficiency is defined as the ratio of cardiac displacement work to the myocardial oxygen consumption. In our experiments the external cardiac work remained unchanged, while myocardial oxygen consumption increased. This fact explains the significant fall in efficiency after thiopentone, methohexitone, Althesin, propanidid, and ketamine and illustrates the uneconomic work of the heart under the influence of these anaesthetic agents. The changes in efficiency after etomidate and piritramide, however, varied within the normal range of error.

The large coronary reserve of a sound heart can compensate even maximum energy requirements. In case of patients with a sound cardiovascular system the choice of the induction agent is, therefore, of minor importance. The myocardial oxygen supply, however, in patients with reduced coronary reserve, hypertension, cardiac insufficiency and shock syndrome, is limited.

Especially after barbiturates, propanidid, and ketamine an additional energy demand during induction of anaesthesia can lead to a disproportion between oxygen supply and oxygen requirement of the heart and thus to a disturbed energy metabolism. Based on this comparative circulatory investigation it is recommended, therefore, in these cases to prefer etomidate or an opiate-type agent, such as piritramide, to the other induction agents under investigation.

Since the hypnotic etomidate has no analgesic properties, while the analgesic piritramide lacks hypnotic properties, it is conceivable that etomidate and piritramide complement each other successfully in a combined anaesthesia.

Summary

The comparative animal experiment was intended to differentiate the acute effects of clinically customary and chemically different intravenous induction agents on haemodynamics, coronary perfusion and myocardial oxygen consumption.

Normoventilated dogs (n = 48) received the following intravenous injections within 25 seconds in a steady-state of a piritramide/N_2O/O_2 basic anaesthesia: methohexitone (2.0 and 4.0 mg/kg; n = 8), thiopentone (5.0 and 10.0 mg/kg; n = 6), propanidid (5.0 and 10.0 mg/kg; n = 8), Althesin (1.0 and 2.0 mg/kg); n = 8)

---

[1] These results are in agreement with EBERLEIN (1966) and KETTLER (1973), who found after barbiturates and ketamine the lowest oxygen saturation in the coronary venous blood as compared with other induction agents.

ketamine (5.0 and 10.0 mg/kg; n = 8), piritramide (0.25 and 0.5 mg/kg; n = 8), and etomidate (0.4 and 0.8 mg/kg; n = 13).

Immediately after the administration of methohexitone, thiopentone Althesin, propanidid, and ketamine the cardiac output (thermodilution method) rose slightly on account of tachycardia, while the peripheral total resistance reacted reversely. The mean arterial pressure only fell noticeably after propanidid and ketamine. The decrease of the stroke volume and the inotropic parameter dp/dt max, as well as the increase in the end-diastolic left ventricular pressure and in the pressure of the pulmonary artery suggest considerable myocardial depressor properties of these anaesthetics. Since external cardiac work remained unchanged and myocardial contractility (dp/dt max) and myocardial wall tension ($\bar{P}_{syst}$) decreased, the increased heart rate alone explains the rise in myocardial oxygen consumption which was met by a coronary perfusion exceeding nutritional requirements (measured with the pressure difference method) after propanidid and Althesin. In the case of barbiturates and ketamine, however, the rise in myocardial oxygen consumption was covered by an increase of coronary blood flow and additional oxygen utilization. Propanidid is, therefore, believed to have an initial coronary dilatory property while the barbiturates and ketamine lead to a constriction of the coronary vessels. The efficiency of cardiac work, defined as the relation between displacement work and energy requirement, decreased and illustrated the uneconomic work of the heart under the influence of these anaesthetic agents. In contrast to the mentioned anaesthetics, etomidate and piritramide did not affect haemodynamics, coronary blood flow and myocardial oxygen consumption during induction.

The comparative circulatory investigations recommend etomidate and/or piritramide as a suitable induction agent for patients with cardiac and coronary insufficiency.

Zusammenfassung

Die vergleichende tierexperimentelle Untersuchung sollte die akuten Wirkungen der klinisch gebräuchlichen, in ihren chemischen Strukturen aber unterschiedlichen, intravenösen Einleitungsanaesthetika auf die Hämodynamik, die Koronarperfusion und den myokardialen Sauerstoffverbrauch näher differenzieren und gegeneinander abgrenzen.

Normoventilierten Hunden (n = 48) wurden im steady-state einer Piritramid/Lachgas/Sauerstoff-Basisnarkose Methohexital (2,0 und 4,0 mg/kg; n = 8), Thiopental (5,0 und 10,0 mg/kg; n = 6), Propanidid (5,0 und 10,0 mg/kg; n = 8), Althesin (1,0 und 2,0 mg/kg; n = 8), Ketamine (5,0 und 10,0 mg/kg; n = 8), Piritramid (0,25 und 0,5 mg/kg; n = 8) und Etomidate (0,4 und 0,8 mg/kg; n = 13) innerhalb von 25 sec intravenös injiziert.
Unmittelbar nach der Applikation von Methohexital, Thiopental, Althesin, Propanidid und Ketamine stieg das Herzzeitvolumen (Thermodilutionsmethode) tachykardiebedingt leicht an, während der periphere Gesamtwiderstand spiegelbildlich zum Verhalten des Herzzeitvolumens abfiel. Der arterielle Mitteldruck fiel nur

nach Propanidid und Ketamin stärker ab. Der Abfall des Schlagvolumens und des Inotropieparameters dp/dt max sowie der Anstieg
des linksventrikulären enddiastolischen Druckes und des Druckes
in der Arteria pulmonalis deuten auf erhebliche myokarddepressive
Eigenschaften dieser Anaesthetika hin. Da die äußere Herzarbeit
unverändert blieb, der kontraktile Zustand des Myokards (dp/dt
max) und die myokardiale Wandspannung $\overline{P}_{syst}$) abfielen, erklärt
der Anstieg der Herzfrequenz allein die Zunahme des myokardialen
Sauerstoffverbrauchs, den nach Propanidid und Althesin eine über
den nutritiven Bedarf hinausgehende Erhöhung der Koronarperfusion
(gemessen mit dem Druckdifferenzverfahren) deckte, während diesen
nach den Barbituraten und Ketaminen eine Zunahme des Koronarflusses
und eine vermehrte Sauerstoffausschöpfung deckte. Der mechanische
Wirkungsgrad für die Herzarbeit, der als Verhältnis zwischen
Verdrängungsarbeit und Energiebedarf definiert ist, fiel ab und
verdeutlichte die unökonomische Arbeit des Herzens unter dem Einfluß dieser Anaesthetika. Im Gegensatz zu den übrigen Anaesthetika
übten Etomidate und Piritramid keinen Einfluß auf die Hämodynamik
und den myokardialen Sauerstoffverbrauch aus.

Die vergleichenden Kreislaufuntersuchungen empfehlen Etomidate
und/oder Piritramid als geeignetes Einleitungsanaesthetikum bei
Patienten mit eingeschränkter kardialer Leistungsbreite.

References

1. VAN ACKERN, K., DEUSTER, J.E., MAST, G.J.: Akute Minderung der Kontrak-
    tilität des Warmblüterorganismus durch Ketamin. Z. prakt. Anaesth.
    Wiederbeleb. 7, 309 (1972).

2. BEER, R., SOGA, D.: Die Beeinflussung der linksventrikulären Myokard-
    kontraktilität und Hämodynamik durch Epontol beim Menschen. Anaesthesist
    20, 480 (1971).

3. BETANCOURT, L.G.: Epontol und Coronardurchblutung. Anaesthesist 19, 48
    (1970).

4. BRETSCHNEIDER, H.J.: Aktuelle Probleme der Koronardurchblutung und des
    Myokardstoffwechsels. Regensburger ärztl. Fortbildung 15, 1 (1967).

5. BRETSCHNEIDER, H.J., COTT, L.A., HENSEL, I., KETTLER, D., MARTEL, J.:
    Ein neuer komplexer hämodynamischer Parameter aus 5 additiven Gliedern
    zur Bestimmung des O_2-Bedarfs des linken Ventrikels. Pflügers Arch.
    ges.Physiol. 319, H.3/4, R 14 (1970).

6. BRETSCHNEIDER, H.J.: Die hämodynamischen Determinanten des O_2-Bedarfs
    des Herzmuskels. Arzneimittel-Forsch. 21, 1515 (1971).

7. BRÜCKNER, J.B., GETHMANN, J.W., PATSCHKE, D., TARNOW, J., WEYMAR, A.:
    Untersuchungen zur Wirkung von Etomidate auf den Kreislauf des Menschen.
    Anaesthesist 23, 322 (1974).

8. DOENICKE, A., LORENZ, W., BEIGL, R., BEZECNY, H., KALMAR, L., PRAETORIUS, B., UHLIG, G.: Histamine release after intravenous application of short-acting hypnotics. A comparison of etomidate, Althesin CT 1341, and propanidid. Brit.J.Anaesth. 45, 1097 (1973).

9. DOENICKE, A., GABANYI, D., LEMCKE, H., SCHURK-BULICH, M.: Kreislaufver-halten und Myokardfunktion nach drei kurzwirkenden i.v. Hypnotika Etomi-date, Propanidid, Methohexital. Anaesthesist 23, 108 (1974).

10. DUDZIAK, R., RAFF, K.W., KOSCHE, F.: Über die Wirkung von Propanidid auf die Coronardurchblutung und Hämodynamik des Hundeherzens. In: Anaesthesio-logie und Wiederbelebung, Bd. 74, S. 51. Berlin-Heidelberg-New York: Springer 1974.

11. EBERLEIN, H.J.: Koronardurchblutung und Sauerstoffversorgung des Herzens unter verschiedenen CO_2-Spannungen und Anaesthetika. Arch. Kreisl.-Forsch. 50, 18 (1966).

12. EGER, E.I., BRANDSTATER, B., SAIDMANN, L.J., REGAN, L.J., SEVERINGHAUS, J.W., MUNSON, E.S.: Equipotent alveolar concentrations of methoxyflurane, halothane, diethyl ether, fluroxene, cyclopropane, xenon und nitrous oxide in the dog. Anesthesiology 26, 771 (1965).

13. EGER, E.I., SAIDMANN, L.J., BRANDSTATER, B.: Minimum alveolar anesthetic concentration: A standard of anesthetic potency. Anesthesiology 26, 756 (1965).

14. FISCHER, K.: Vergleichende tierexperimentelle Untersuchungen zum Einfluß verschiedener Narkotika auf das Herz. In: Ketamin (Ed. M. Gemperle, H. Kreuscher, D. Langrehr), S. 11. Anaesthesiologie und Wiederbelebung, Bd. 69. Berlin-Heidelberg-New York: Springer 1973.

15. GEMPERLE, M., MORET, P., MEGEVAND, R.: Neuroleptanalgesie et système cardiovasculaire. Ann. Anesth. franç. VII, Spécial 1, 87 (1966).

16. GODEFROI, E.F., JANSSEN, P.A.J., VAN DER EYCKEN, C.A.M., VAN HEERTUM, A.H.M.T., NIEMEGEERS, C.J.E.: DL-1 (1 Arylalkyl) imidazole-5-carboxylate Esters, a novel type of hypnotic agents. J. Med. chem. Pharm. Chem. 8, 320 (1965).

17. GOLDSTEIN, A. jr., KEATS, A.S.: The risk of anaesthesia. Anesthesiology 33, 130 (1970).

18. GREGG, D.E., FISCHER, L.C.: Blood supply to the heart. Handbook of Physiology. Washington: Amer. Physiol. Soc. (1963).

19. HEISS, H.W., HENSEL, I., KETTLER, D., TAUCHERT, M., BRETSCHNEIDER, H.J.: Über den Anteil des Koronarsinus-Ausflusses an der Myokarddurchblutung des linken Ventrikels. Z. Kardiol. 62, 593 (1973).

20. HEITMANN, H.B., DRECHSEL, U., HERPFER, G., ZINDLER, M.: Die Wirkung von Piritramid (Dipidolor) auf die Regulation der Atmung und die orthostatische Stabilität des Kreislaufs. Anaesthesist 19, 152 (1970).

21. HEMPELMANN, G., KETTLER, D., HOLZHÄUSER, H., HEMPELMANN, W., HENSEL, I., KARLICZEK, G., KIRCHNER, E.: Kombination von Piritramid und N_2O - ein neues Narkoseverfahren. Teil II: Untersuchungen am Menschen. Z. prakt. Anaesth. Wiederbeleb. 6, 339 (1971).

22. HENSEL, I., BRETSCHNEIDER, H.J.: Pitot-Rohr-Katheter für die fortlaufende Messung der Koronar- und Nierendurchblutung im Tierexperiment. Arch. Kreisl.-Forsch. 62, 249 (1970).

23. HENSEL, I., BRAUN, U., KETTLER, D., KNOLL, D., MARTEL, J., PASCHEN, K.: Untersuchungen über die Kreislauf- und Stoffwechselveränderungen unter Ketamin-Narkose. Anaesthesist 21, 44 (1972).

24. JANSSEN, P.A.J., NIEMEGEERS, C.J.E., SCHELLEKENS, K.H.L., LENAERTS, F.M.: Etomidate, R-(+)-Ethyl-1-(α methyl-benzyl) imidazole-5-carboxylate (R 16 659) a potent, short-acting relatively atoxic intravenous hypnotic agent in rats. Arzneim.-Forsch. 21, 1234 (1971).

25. KETTLER, D.: Hämodynamische Komponenten des myokardialen Energiebedarfs und Sauerstoffversorgung des Herzens bei verschiedenen Narkosen. Anaesthesiologie und Wiederbelebung, Bd. 67. Berlin-Heidelberg-New York: Springer 1973.

26. KETTLER, D., BRAUN, U., COTT, L.A., HEISS, H.W., HENSEL, I., MARTEL, J., PASCHEN, K., BRETSCHNEIDER, H.J.: Kombination von Piritramid und N_2O - ein neues Narkoseverfahren Teil I: Tierexperimentelle Untersuchungen. Z. prakt. Anaesth. Wiederbeleb. 6, 329 (1971).

27. KETTLER, D., SONNTAG, H., DONATH, K., REGENSBURGER, D., SCHENK, H.D.: Hämodynamik, Myokardmechanik, Sauerstoffbedarf und Sauerstoffversorgung des menschlichen Herzens mit Etomidate. Anaesthesist 23, 116 (1974).

28. LOCHNER, W.: Herz, In: Physiologie des Kreislaufs, Bd. 1 (Ed. E. Bauereisen), S. 195. Berlin-Heidelberg-New York: Springer 1971

29. LUTZ, H., PETER, K., JUHRAN, W.: Hämodynamische Reaktionen nach Anwendung von Ketamin. Z. prakt. Anaesth. Wiederbeleb. 7, 8 (1972).

30. MAAS, A.H.J., HEMELINK, M.L., DE LEEUV, R.J.M.: An evaluation of the spectrophotometric determination of $Hb-O_2$, Hb-CO and Hb in blood with the CO-oximeter IL 182. Clin. chim. Acta 29, 303 (1970).

31. MASON, D.T.: Usefulness and limitations of the rate of rise of intraventricular pressure (dp/dt) in the evaluation of myocardial contractility in man. Amer.J.Cardiol. 23, 516 (1969).

32. MONTEL, H., STARKE, K., SCHÜRMANN, H.J.: Tierexperimentelle Untersuchungen zum Mechanismus der pulsfrequenz- und blutdrucksteigernden Wirkung des Ketamins. In: Ketamin (Ed. M. Gemperle, H. Kreuscher, D. Langrehr), S. 77. Anaesthesiologie und Wiederbelebung Bd. 69. Berlin-Heidelberg-New York: Springer 1973.

33. MUSCHOLL, E.: Diskussionsbeitrag in: Ketamin (Ed. M. Gemperle, H. Kreuscher, D. Langrehr), S. 178. Anaesthesiologie und Wiederbelebung, Bd. 69. Berlin-Heidelberg-New York: Springer 1973.

34. O'ROURKE, R.A., BISHOP, V.S.: Cardiovascular hemodynamics in the conscious dog. Amer. Heart J. 81, 55 (1971).

35. ROWE. G.G.: Responses of the coronary circulation to physiologic changes and pharmacologic agents. Anesthesiology 41, 182 (1974).

36. SCHORER, R.: Die Technik der Thermo-Injektionsmethode mit Direktanzeige zur Bestimmung des Herzzeitvolumens. Z. prakt. Anaesth. Wiederbeleb. 2, 28 (1967).

37. SEVERINGHAUS, J.W.: Role of lung factors. In: Uptake and distribution of anesthetic agents (Ed. E.M. Papper, R.J. Kitz), p. 59. New York → Toronto — London: McGraw-Hill: 1962.

38. SIEGEL, H.J., SONNENBLICK, E.H., JUDGE, D., WILSON, W.S.: The quantification of myocardial contractility in dog and man. Cardiologica 45, 189 (1964).

39. SLAMA, H., PIIPER, J.: Direktanzeigendes Rechengerät zur Bestimmung des Herzzeitvolumens mit der Thermoinjektionsmethode. Z. Kreisl.-Forsch. 53, 322 (1964).

40. SOGA, D., BEER, R.: Myocardkontraktilität und Hämodynamik im Verlauf einer Methohexital-Narkose. Anaesthesiologie und Wiederbelebung, Bd. 57. Berlin-Heidelberg-New York: Springer 1972

41. SOGA, D., BEER, R.: Myokardkontraktilität und Narkose. Anaesthesist 21, 165 (1972).

42. SONNTAG, H.: Koronardurchblutung und Energieumsatz des menschlichen Herzens unter verschiedenen Anaesthetika. Anaesthesiologie und Wiederbelebung, Bd. 79. Berlin-Heidelberg-New York: Springer 1974.

43. SONNTAG, H., SCHENK, H.D., REGENSBURGER, D., KETTLER, D., HELLBERG, K., KNOLL, D., DONATH, U., BECKER, H.: Effects of Althesin (Glaxo CT 1341) on Coronary Blood Flow and Myocardial Metabolism in Man. Acta anaesth. scand. 17, 218 (1973).

44. SMITH, G., VANCE, J.P., BROWN, D.M.: The effect of propanidid on myocardial blood flow and oxygen consumption in the dog. Brit. J. Anaesth. 45, 691 (1973).

45. STRAUER, B.E.: Contractile responses to morphine, meperidine, piritramide and fentanyl: A comparative study on the isolated ventricular myocardium. Anesthesiology 37, 304 (1972).

46. SZAPPANOS, G., BEAUMANOIR, A., GEMPERLE, G., GEMPERLE M., MORET, P.: The effect of ketamine on the cardiovascular and central nervous system (Ed. H. Kreuscher). Anaesthesiologie und Wiederbelebung, Bd. 40. Berlin-Heidelberg-New York: Springer 1969.

47. TRABER, D.L., WILSON, R.D., PRIANO, L.L.: Blockade of the hypertensive response to ketamine. Anaesth. Analg. Curr. Res. 49, 420 (1970).

48. WALLACE, A.G., SKINNER, N.S., MITCHELL, J.H.: Haemodynamic determinants of the maximal rate of rise of left ventricular pressure. Amer. J. Physiol. 205, 30 (1963).

49. WEYMAR, A., EIGENHEER, F., GETHMANN, J.W., REINECKE, A., PATSCHKE, D., TARNOW, J., BRÜCKNER, J.B.: Tierexperimentelle Untersuchungen zur Wirkung von Etomidate (R 26 490-Sulfat) auf den Kreislauf und die myokardiale Sauerstoffversorgung. Anaesthesist 23, 150 (1974).

50. WIRTH, W., HOFFMEISTER, F.: Pharmakologische Untersuchungen mit Propanidid. In: Horatz, K., Frey, R., Zindler, M.: Die intravenöse Kurznarkose mit dem neuen Phenoxyessigsäurederivat Propanidid (Epontol). Anaesthesiologie und Wiederbelebung, Bd. 4. Berlin-Heidelberg-New York: Springer 1965.

Haemodynamic Effects of Etomidate - a New Hypnotic - in Patients with Myocardial Insufficiency

G. Hempelmann, W. Oster, S. Piepenbrock and G. Karliczek

Introduction

Since the introduction of etomidate by JANSSEN et al. (1971) and the first clinical reports by DOENICKE et al. (1973 a-e, 1974) there has been much interest in this new imidazole-carboxylate hypnotic. All of the clinical investigations have been performed in volunteers or patients with a normal cardiovascular system (BRÜCKNER et al., 1974; KETTLER et al., 1974). In these patients etomidate had only little influence on haemodynamic parameters.

Material and Method

It was our interest to see, whether or not etomidate had any more marked effect on haemodynamics in patients with myocardial disease. Therefore, this hypnotic has been given to a total of 34 patients with heart diseases, all functional class III.

Group 1: After sternotomy and pericardiotomy in neuroleptanalgesia, muscle relaxation and controlled ventilation with 40 % oxygen and 60 % nitrous oxide on-line registration of the following haemo- dynamic parameters has been carried out in 13 patients, age 24 - 59 years (mean 46.3 years) (Fig. 1): Electrocardiogram with heart rate monitoring, arterial blood pressure in a radial artery using Statham transducers, left ventricular pressure, dp/dt - the first derivative of left ventricular pressure, left ventricular enddia- stolic pressure, and central venous pressure. The left ventricle was punctured using a steel needle, which had been connected to a Statham transducer SP 37 (HEMPELMANN et al., 1973). After heparinisation - by the way, heparin is not having any relevant haemodynamic effect - etomidate was given intravenously in a dose of 0.3 mg/kg within 15 seconds.

Group 2: In another group of 12 patients, age 37 - 68 years, mean 49.4 years, we investigated the effect of 0.3 mg/kg etomidate on the vascular system during extracorporeal circulation. In these patients ventricular fibrillation was induced electrically as part of the surgical procedure. With the heart not beating, the aorta crossclamped, a volume-constant perfusion-flow of the pump oxygenator and no changes in blood temperature, blood gases and acid-base parameters, any change in arterial pressure can be attributed to a change in vascular tone or total peripheral resistance.

Group 3: 1 - 3 hours following cardiac surgery in extracorporeal circulation we have performed some more haemodynamic investi- gations in 9 patients, age 19 - 49 years, mean 38.6 years.

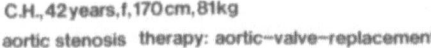

C.H., 42 years, f, 170 cm, 81 kg

aortic stenosis therapy: aortic-valve-replacement

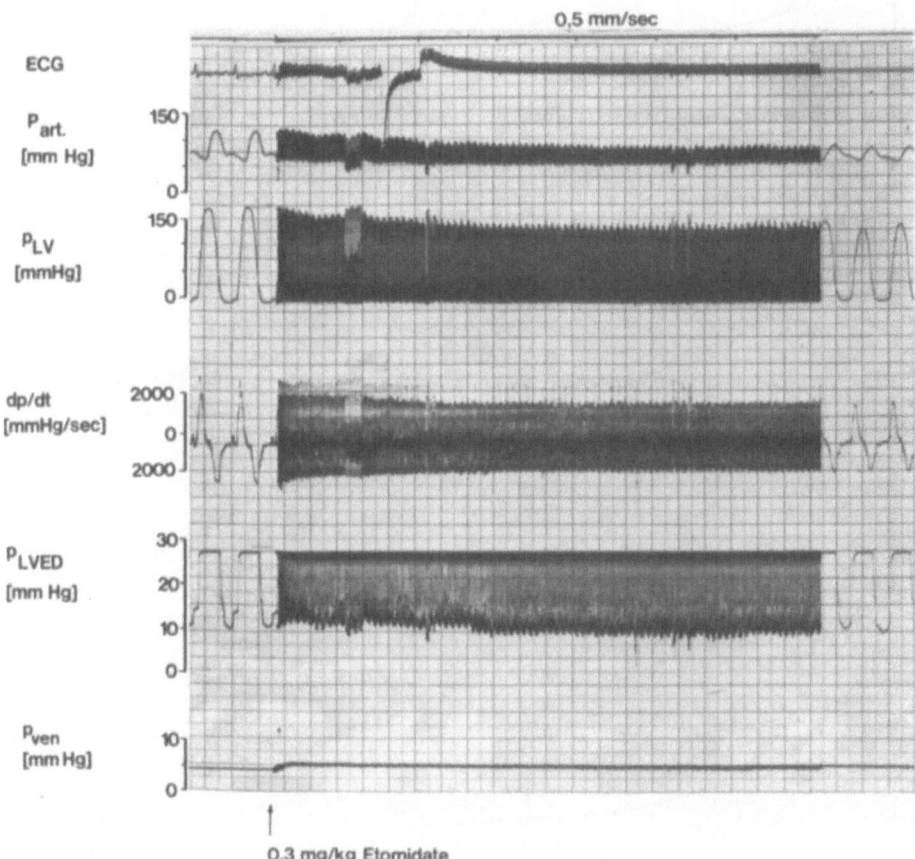

Fig. 1.Haemodynamic changes after injection of 0.3 mg/kg etomidate in a patient with aortic stenosis

Before and for a period of 15 minutes following injection of 0.3 mg/kg etomidate, arterial blood pressure, right and left atrial pressures, heart rate, and cardiac output were monitored. The thermodilution technique was used for cardiac output measurements with injection of cold saline solution ($0 - 4^\circ$C) into the left atrium and on-line registration of dilution curves by a thermistor placed into the thoracic aorta via a femoral-artery-catheter (HEMPELMANN et al., 1972).

Results

The haemodynamic results of group 1 are summed up in Fig. 2:

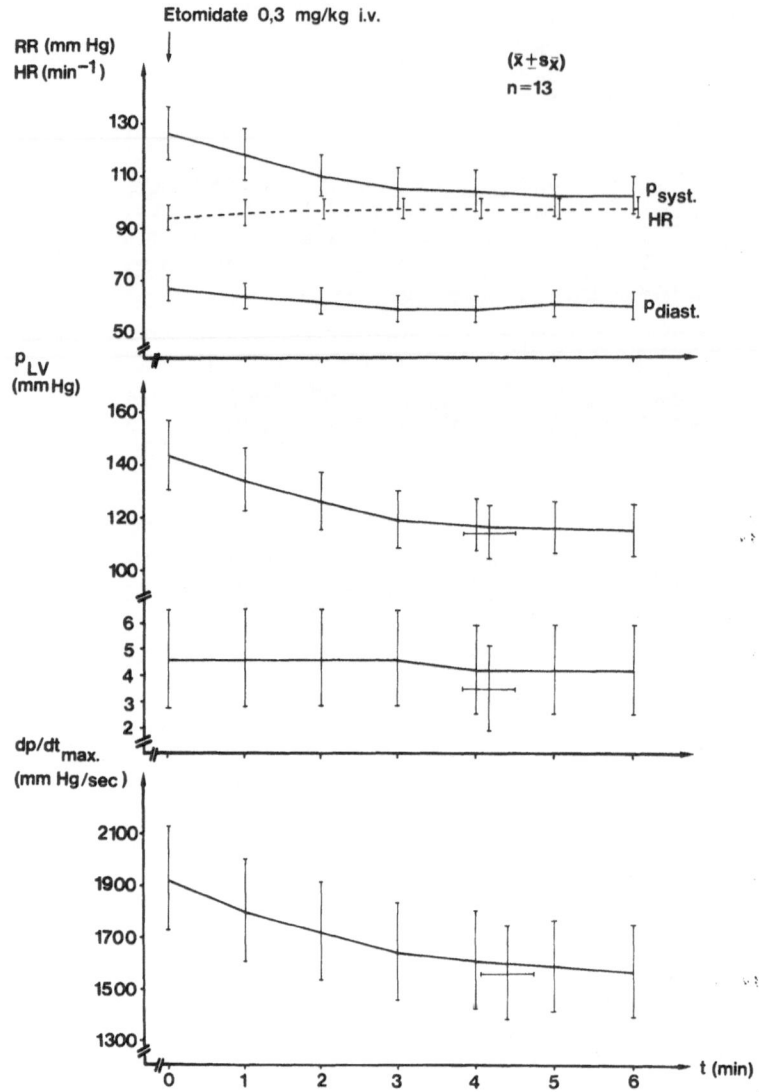

Fig. 2.Changes in blood pressure (RR), heart rate (HR), left ventricular pressure (p_{LV}), and the first derivative of left ventricular pressure (dp/dt_{max}) after injection of 0.3 mg/kg etomidate in patients with myocardial diseases

There were only minor changes in heart rate (control value 94 beats per minute). Six minutes after application of etomidate there was a significant decrease in systolic pressure and left ventricular pressure of 20 % each. Mean arterial blood pressure decreased by 15 %. Simultaneous registration of dp/dt demonstrated an 18 % decrease in this left ventricular contractility parameter.

Changes in left ventricular enddiastolic pressure and central venous pressure were only small and statistically not significant.

Fig. 3 is showing an original pressure-recording during extra-corporeal circulation (group 2): In this patient 0.3 mg/kg etomi-date was injected intravenously; perfusion pressure - measured via Statham transducer in the left radial artery - went down as a result of etomidate-induced vasodilation.

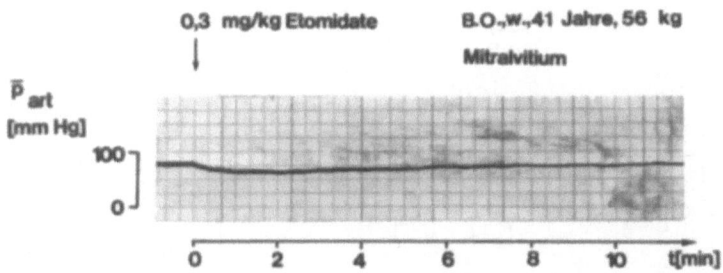

Fig. 3.Changes in perfusion pressure during extracorporeal circulation in a patient with mitral valve disease after injection of 0.3 mg/kg etomidate

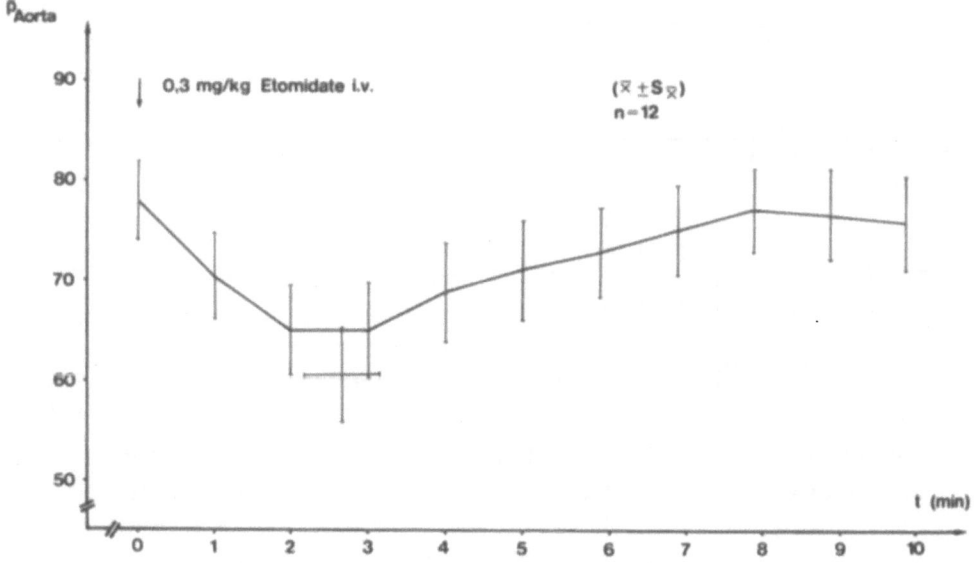

Fig. 4.Mean changes in perfusion pressure during extracorporeal circulation in 12 patients with heart diseases

Mean changes in this group of 12 patients are shown in Fig. 4:
0.3 mg/kg etomidate caused a decrease in perfusion pressure from
77.9 ± 4.1 mm Hg to a minimum, which was 22 % below control values.
Eight minutes after i.v. injection perfusion pressure was back
to control values.

In group 3   0.3 mg/kg etomidate decreased systolic blood pressure
by - 10 %, diastolic blood pressure by - 7 %, and increased heart
rate by + 3 %, which is in accordance with the results in our
first group of patients (Fig. 5).

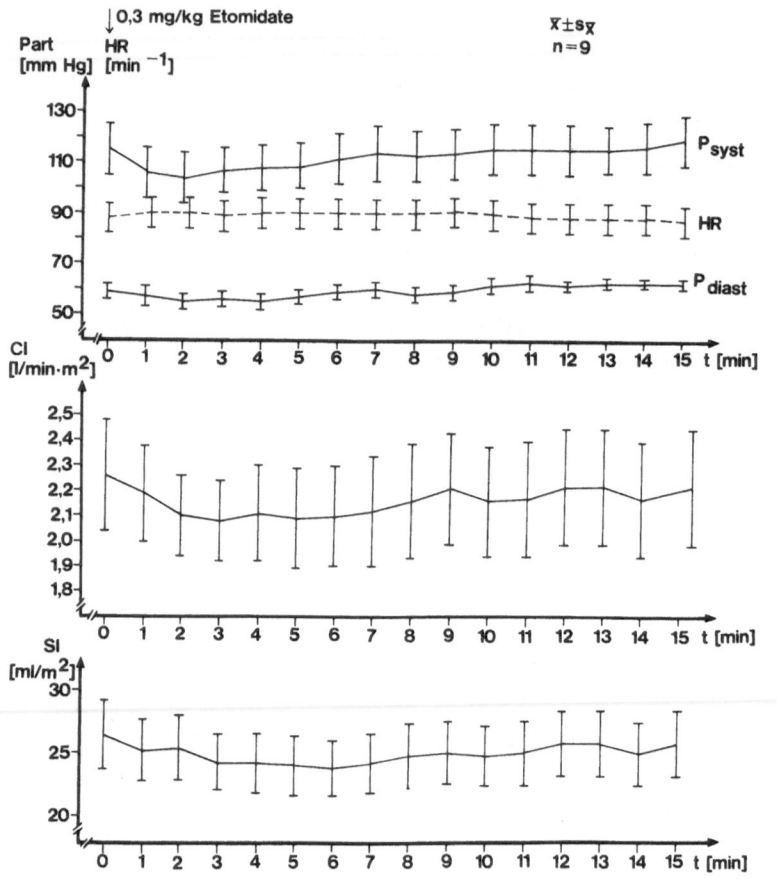

Fig. 5.Mean changes in arterial pressure (p_{art}), heart rate (HR), cardiac
index (CI), and stroke index (SI) after injection of 0.3 mg/kg etomidate

Cardiac index decreased initially from a mean of 2.26 ± 0.22
1/min · m^2 to a minimum of 2.08 ± 0.16 1/min · m^2 (- 8 %) three
minutes after injection of the hypnotic. Control values were
reached again after approx. 9 minutes. Stroke index decreased
by - 10 %; here control values were reached again after 12 min.

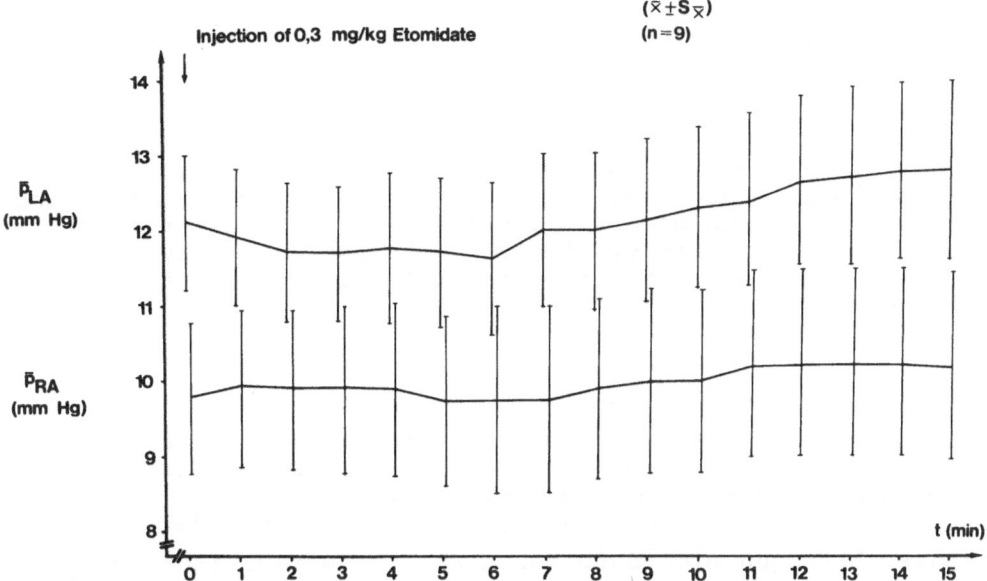

Fig. 6. Mean changes in right and left atrial pressure after injection of etomidate (0.3 mg/kg) in patients with myocardial diseases

There were only minor changes in left and right atrial pressure (Fig. 6). Total peripheral resistance initially decreased and then increased by 9 % up to the 15th minute.

Discussion

Our haemodynamic investigations in a total of 34 patients with heart diseases, functional class III demonstrate, that 0.3 mg/kg etomidate has a moderate effect on haemodynamic parameters, comparable to 1 mg/kg methohexitone for example. The decrease in dp/dt$_{max}$ with almost no change in heart rate and left ventricular enddiastolic pressure confirms that etomidate has a negative inotropic effect; this is, however, less than with Althesin, propanidid or thiopental (HEMPELMANN et al., 1974), which is in accordance with results by BRÜCKNER et al., (1974). KETTLER et al., (1974) reported on positive inotropic effects of etomidate in patients with normal cardiovascular systems. Recently, however, they mentioned similar negative inotropic effects in 3 patients with severe myocardial lesions (KETTLER et al., 1974).

Our results of cardiac index and stroke index calculation confirm, that etomidate has a negative inotropic effect. Compared to thiopental (- 34 %) or propanidid (- 40 %) the decrease in cardiac index, however, is small (HEMPELMANN, 1973). Changes in perfusion pressure during extracorporeal circulation demonstrated, that etomidate has a vasodilating effect as well. Both effects -

vasodilation and negative inotropy - seem to be similar percentage-wise. In contrast, enflurane, e.g., has a more marked effect on the myocardium (KARLICZEK et al., 1974).

The new hypnotic etomidate has lesser haemodynamic effects compared to other short-acting induction agents such as methohexitone, Althesin, propanidid or thiopental (HEMPELMANN et al., 1974). Therefore, we think that etomidate can be used safely for induction of anaesthesia, e.g. neuroleptanalgesia, especially in patients with myocardial insufficiency. Etomidate, however, is only a hypnotic without any analgetic effect; it therefore cannot be used as a mononarcotic.

Summary

The new hypnotic etomidate has been investigated in a total of 34 patients using 0.3 mg/kg b.w. There were only minor changes in arterial pressure, heart rate, left ventricular pressure, left ventricular enddiastolic pressure, dp/dt_{max}, cardiac index and stroke index. Although etomidate has a small negative inotropic effect in patients with myocardial insufficiency (dp/dt_{max} - 18 %), we think that it is of great value especially in this group of patients for induction of anaesthesia.

Zusammenfassung

Das neue Hypnotikum Etomidate wurde an insgesamt 34 Patienten in einer Dosierung von 0,3 mg/kg erprobt, wobei nur geringfügige Veränderungen des Blutdrucks, der Herzfrequenz, des linksventrikulären Drucks, des linksventrikulären enddiastolischen Drucks, der maximalen Druckanstiegsgeschwindigkeit, des Herz- und Schlagindex festgestellt werden konnten. Obwohl Etomidate bei den von uns untersuchten Patienten mit myocardialem Vorschaden eine geringe negativ inotrope Wirkung zeigte (dp/dt_{max} - 18 %), möchten wir dieser Substanz - insbesondere bei myokardialen Risikopatienten - eine besondere Stellung, z.B. bei der Narkoseeinleitung, einräumen.

References

1. BRÜCKNER J.B., GETHMANN, J.W., PATSCHKE, D., TARNOW, J., WEYMAR, A.: Untersuchungen zur Wirkung von Etomidate auf den Kreislauf des Menschen. Anaesthesist 23, 322 (1974).

2. DOENICKE, A.: Klinisch-experimentelle Untersuchungen und klinischer Erfahrungsbericht über ein neues i.v. applizierbares Narkotikum. 6. Internationaler Fortbildungskurs für klinische Anaesthesiologie, Wien, 21.-25. Mai 1973. Tagungsbericht.

3. DOENICKE, A., KUGLER, J., PENZEL, G., LAUB, M., KALMAR., J., KILLIAN, I., BEZECNY, H.: Hirnfunktion und Toleranzbreite nach Etomidate, einem neuen barbituratfreien i.v. applizierbaren Hypnotikum. Anaesthesist 22., 357 (1973).

4. DOENICKE, A., KALMAR, L.: Die Aufgaben des Anaesthesisten bei der Erprobung neuer Anaesthetica. Wandertagung; Ungarische Gesellschaft für Anaesthesiologie und Reanimation, Debrecen, August 1973. Tagungsbericht.

5. DOENICKE, A., KUGLER, J., LORENZ, W., WAGNER, E., BEZECNY, H., BAUER, I., DENFFER, I., KALMAR, L., PRAETORIUS, B., SCHELLENBERGER, A., SCHUNDINGER, St., SPIESS, W.: Experimentelle Untersuchungen und klinische Erfahrungen mit dem neuen i.v. Kurznarkotikum Etomidate. Vortrag XIII. Gemeinsame Tagung der Deutschen, Schweizerischen und Österreichischen Gesellschaften für Anaesthesiologie und Reanimation, Linz, September 1973. Anaesthesiologie und Wiederbelebung, Bd. 93. Berlin-Heidelberg-New York: Springer, 1975.

6. DOENICKE, A., WAGNER, E., BEETZ, K.H.: Blutgasanalysen (arteriell) nach drei kurzwirksamen i.v. Hypnotika (Propanidid, Etomidate, Methohexital). Anaesthesist $\underline{22}$, 353 (1973).

7. DOENICKE, A., GABANYI, D., LEMCKE, H., SCHÜRK-BULICH, M.: Kreislaufverhalten und Myocardfunktion nach drei kurzwirksamen i.v. Hypnotika: Etomidate, Propanidid, Methohexital. Anaesthesist $\underline{23}$, 108 (1974).

8. HEMPELMANN, G.: Respiratorische und hämodynamische Probleme im anaesthesiologischen Bereich. Ergebnisse der fortlaufenden Sauerstoffpartialdruckmessung im Blut sowie der Herzzeitvolumen-Bestimmung mit der Kälteverdünnungsmethode. Habilitationsschrift, Hannover 1973.

9. HEMPELMANN, G., HELMS, U., WALDHAUSEN, E., DALICHAU, H., WALTER, P., PIEPENBROCK, S.: Kreislaufuntersuchungen über CT 1341 bei Patienten mit angeborenen und erworbenen Herzfehlern. Anaesthesist $\underline{22}$, 345 (1973).

10. HEMPELMANN, G., HEMPELMANN, W., PIEPENBROCK, S., OSTER, W., KARLICZEK, G.: Die Beeinflussung der Blutgase und Hämodynamik durch Etomidate bei myokardial vorgeschädigten Patienten. Anaesthesist $\underline{23}$, 423 (1974).

11. HEMPELMANN, G., KARLICZEK, G., HELMS, U., HEMPELMANN, W.: Akute hämodynamische Veränderungen durch tracheobronchiales Absaugen. Z. Kreisl.-Forsch. $\underline{61}$, 545 (1972).

12. HEMPELMANN, G., KARLICZEK, G., PIEPENBROCK, S.: Hämodynamische Untersuchungen bei über 100 herzchirurgischen Patienten unter Verwendung von 10 verschiedenen Narkoseverfahren. DGAW Jahrestagung 1974, Kongreßband, Erlangen: Perimed, 1975.

13. JANSSEN, P.A.J., NIEMEGEERS, C.J.E., SCHELLEKENS, K.H.L., LENAERTS, F.M.: Etomidate, R(+)Ethyl-1-(alpha-methyl-benzyl)imidazole-5-carboxylate (R 16659), a potent, short acting relatively atoxic intravenous hypnotic agent in rats. Arzneimittel-Forsch. $\underline{21}$, 1234 (1971).

14. KARLICZEK, G., HEMPELMANN, G., PIEPENBROCK, S., BÜTER, F.: Die Beeinflussung der Hämodynamik durch Enflurane bei myokardial vorgeschädigten Patienten. Anaesthesist $\underline{23}$, 490 (1974).

15. KETTLER, D., SONNTAG, H., DONATH, U., REGENSBURGER, D., SCHENK, H.D.: Hämodynamik, Myocardmechanik, Sauerstoffbedarf und Sauerstoffversorgung des menschlichen Herzens unter Narkoseeinleitung mit Etomidate. Anaesthesist $\underline{23}$, 116 (1974).

16. KETTLER, D., SONNTAG, H.: Hämodynamik bei Patienten mit Herzklappenfeh-
    lern unter Narkoseeinleitung mit Etomidate. Mitteilung, 3. Etomidate-
    Kolloquium in Berlin, 8.2.1974.

Haemodynamics, Myocardial Function, Oxygen Requirement, and Oxygen Supply of the Human Heart after Administration of Etomidate[+]

D. Kettler, H. Sonntag, U. Wolfram-Donath, H.J. Hoeft,
D. Regensburger and H.D. Schenk

In recent years a number of new intravenous anaesthetics have been developed, most of which do not belong to the group of barbiturates, and which raised great hopes with regard to their less pronounced effects on respiration and circulation. Some examples are the preparations used in neuroleptanalgesia (NLA), propanidid, ketamine, the steroid anaesthetic Althesin, and the new short-acting barbiturate methohexital.

After varying periods of enthusiasm, however, objective tests showed that all these new pharmacological developments affect the cardiovascular system (in some cases considerably), and can lead to serious complications, particularly in patients with reduced cardiovascular reserve. Without going into detail, we can mention here the drop in blood pressure after propanidid, Althesin, and droperidol and undesirable increases in blood pressure and heart rate after ketamine.

d-etomidate, which has been developed by Janssen Pharmaceutica, Beerse (Belgium), is a new non-barbiturate preparation with a merely hypnotic action that is still at the stage of animal experimentation and clinical trials.

According to JANSSEN, etomidate differs from other intravenous anaesthetics mainly in having a considerably greater safety margin (6). Extensive initial investigations on human subjects have been carried out by DOENICKE et al. (3) and have shown that etomidate causes only insignificant changes in the respiratory and cardiovascular functions.

A number of investigators (2, 4, 5, 16) have confirmed that etomidate produces only small respiratory and circulatory side effects in animals and in man.

We have therefore included this preparation in our investigation project "Effects of Intravenous Anaesthetics on Heart and Circulation", which has been in progress for a number of years. The advantage of longterm comparative studies of this type lies in the preplanned course of the investigation, which is the same for all the preparations examined and is repeated as matter of routine. Details of the results obtained so far can be found in the monograph by SONNTAG (10) and further publications by our research staff (7, 8, 11, 12, 13, 14, 15).

[+]With the support of Deutsche Forschungsgemeinschaft within the SFB 89-Kardiologie, Göttingen

The aim of this investigation was to examine the effects of etomidate on the general and coronary haemodynamics, the myocardial function, and the oxygen requirement of the left ventricle in human subjects. Up to now the anaesthetics Althesin, ketamine, methohexital, propanidid, thiopental as well as the components of the neuroleptanalgesia (droperidol and fentanyl) and finally etomidate have been studied.

Methods

Preliminary investigations were carried out on dogs. Thereafter, studies were also performed on a total of 5 patients with no heart or circulatory disorders who were undergoing thoracic or vascular surgery. All the patients received a detailed explanation of the proposed investigation and gave their written consent. To prevent the action of etomidate from being influenced by other pharmacological effects, no premedication was given.

After a sleep-inducing dose of 0.3 mg of etomidate/kg wt. i.v., the duration of sleep was extended to about 10 min by a further injection or by a continuous infusion of etomidate. The average dose of etomidate was 0.12 mg/kg · min. After the 10-minute investigation period, the immobilized patients were intubated and artificially ventilated.
Anaesthesia was continued by neuroleptanalgesia. Analysis of the circulation had been carried out as control before etomidate injection. The necessary catheterization was carried out under local anaesthesia with X-ray monitoring. The measurements under etomidate were started about 2-3 min after the induction of sleep, when the circulation had become stabile, and lasted about 6 min.

The following parameters were checked before and under the action of etomidate and recorded on a 6-channel UV recorder: (Fig. 1)

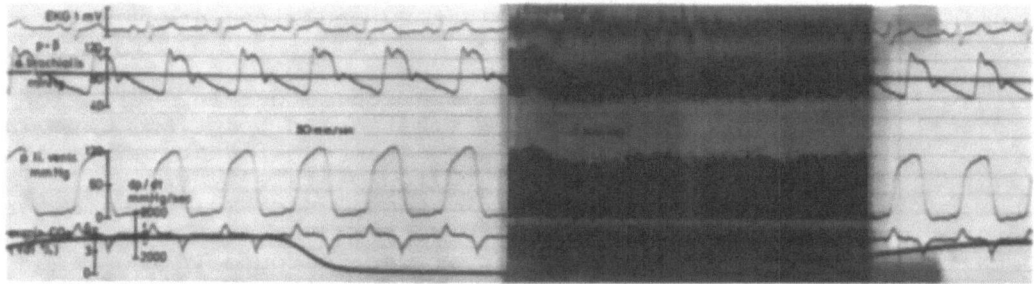

Fig. 1.Haemodynamic effects of 0.3 mg/kg etomidate in man. Recordings from top to bottom: ECG (lead II), arterial (including mean) pressure, left ventricular pressure, rate of left ventricular pressure rise (dp/dt) and expiratory CO_2. Etomidate causes a mild and transitory drop of the arterial pressures

ECG (lead II), arterial pressure including mean pressure, left
ventricular pressure (catheter tip manometer) and rate of pressure
rise (dp/dt), as well as the endexperiratory CO_2 content.

At the same time the cardiac output (CO) was determined by thermodilution (SLAMA-PIIPER method). The O_2 contents of the arterial
and the coronary venous blood (CO-Oximeter), the blood gases, the
acid-base equilibrium, and the serum electrolytes were also
measured. No significant changes were found in the latter parameters. They are therefore not reproduced here.

Coronary blood flow (MBF) was measured by BRETSCHNEIDER's argon
inert-gas method; this and other particulars of the methods used
are described in detail elsewhere (7). The experimental results
were used for additional calculation of the coronary (CVR) and
total peripheral resistance (TPR), the cardiac index (CI), the
stroke volume index (SVI), and the oxygen consumption of the left
ventricle ($M\dot{V}O_2$).

In a second part of the study 10 patients suffering from mitral
or aortic heart valve disease (New York Heart Association classification stage III-IV) and scheduled for valve replacement were
studied. In order to avoid negative side effects these patients
were premedicated with 5 mg droperidol, 0.1 mg fentanyl and
0.5 mg atropine and received an additional dose of $1.5 \mu g/kg$
fentanyl i.v. 2 min prior to injection of 0.3 mg/kg etomidate.
Analyses were carried out after fentanyl and etomidate as well.
In this group no measurements of MBF, $M\dot{V}O_2$ and left ventricular
pressures were performed, in order to keep the risk as low as
possible. Only in 4 out of the 10 patients cardiac output was
determined.
The mean ($\bar{x}$) and the standard error of the mean ($s_{\bar{x}}$) were calculated from the individual values. The t-test of the paired
differences was used as a statistical method for significance
evaluation.

Results

First Part of the Study
General Reactions

After injection of etomidate, falling asleep occurred quickly
and without complications. After the operation, none of the
patients had any unpleasant recollections. However, 4 of the 5
patients developed pronounced myocloni (tightening of the arms
and legs, to-and-fro movements of the hands) under the action
of etomidate, and this made measurements very difficult. Though
some of the patients had to be held down on the examination table,
no excitatory circulation reactions occured. All the patients
showed strong motor reactions to pain stimuli (e.g. pinpricks).
Anisocoria together with dilation and loss of roundness of the
pupils were often observed. It was not possible to eliminate
these effects by further increase of the dose of etomidate.

In the second part of the study premedication with droperidol and fentanyl and an i.v. injection of 1.5 μg/kg fentanyl prior to the application of etomidate were able to prevent all these undesired side effects [+].

General Cardiovascular Effects

In preliminary investigations on dogs, the injection of etomidate in a dose of 0.15 mg/kg during a piritramide-N_2O/O_2 anaesthesia led to a "calming" of the circulation and a slight decrease in the aortic pressures. The O_2 consumption of the heart, as determined by the complex parameter given by BRETSCHNEIDER et al. ($\underline{1}$), decreased slightly. (Fig. 2)

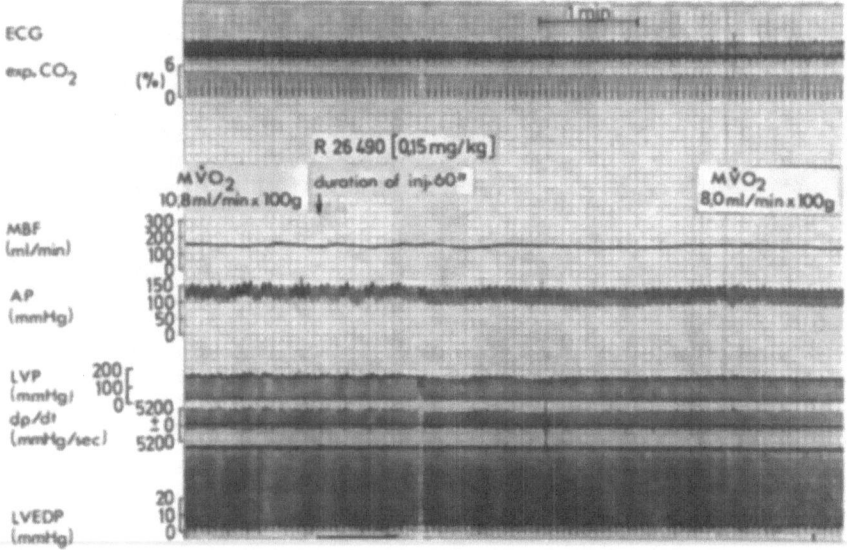

Fig. 2. *Effect of 0.15 mg/kg etomdiate in the artificially ventilated anaesthetized dog (piritramide-N_2O/O_2-anaesthesia) on the ECG (lead II), expiratory CO_2, myocardial blood flow (MBF), myocardial O_2 consumption, aortic (AP) and left ventricular (LVP) pressure, dp/dt and left ventricular enddiastolic pressure (LVEDP). $M\dot{V}O_2$ is calculated from haemodynamic variables by means of the complex parameter after BRETSCHNEIDER et al ($\underline{1}$)*

[+] Premedication with Thalamonal (droperidol and fentanyl) and atropine as well as a previous injection of fentanyl is, therefore, at present our standard technique when induction of anaesthesia with etomidate is planned.

The experimental results of the clinical tests are presented in Table 1. On the whole, the various circulatory parameters were not appreciably influenced by etomidate. The changes in the mean arterial (MAP) pressure, the stroke volume index (SVI), the left ventricular enddiastolic pressure (LVEDP), and dp/dt_{max} are statistically not significant at the 5 % level. The heart rate showed a slight increase of 9 % ($p < 0.01$). While the stroke volume remained unchanged, the cardiac index (CI) increased by 14 % ($p < 0.01$) with a corresponding decrease in the peripheral resistance.

Table 1. Effects of 0.12 mg/kg min etomidate on the haemodynamics in 5 patients without circulatory disease. No premedication. Mean ($\bar{x}$) and S.E.M. ($s_{\bar{x}}$). MAP = mean arterial pressure, HR = heart rate, CI = cardiac index, SVI = stroke volume index, TPR = total peripheral resistance, dp/dt_{max} = maximal rate of left ventric. pressure rise, LVEDP = left ventric. enddiastolic pressure

		Control		Etomidate		Change (%)
		x	$s_{\bar{x}}$	x	$s_{\bar{x}}$	
MAP	mm Hg	92	2	90	2	−
HR	1/min	81	4	88[a]	4	+ 9
CI	$1/min \cdot m^2$	3.44	0.17	3.93[a]	0.15	+ 14
SVI	ml/m^2	43	3	45	4	−
TPR	$\frac{mm\ Hg}{ml/min \cdot kg}$	1.05	0.11	0.92[a]	0.09	− 12
dp/dt_{max}	mm Hg/sec	1163	49	1178	38	−
LVEDP	mm Hg	11.0	0.4	10.9	0.2	−

[a] $p < 0,01$

Coronary Haemodynamics and Myocardial Oxygen Consumption (Table 2)

The coronary perfusion pressure ($\bar{p}$ diast) was unchanged under the influence of etomidate. The pattern of the O_2 supply of the heart with etomidate is different from that of the other anaesthetics investigated (cf. Table 3). The arterio-coronary venous O_2 difference (AVD-O_2) decreased while the coronary blood flow (MBF) increased by 19 % ($p < 0.025$), with a corresponding decrease in the coronary resistance (CVR).

The most important parameter in this table, the myocardial oxygen consumption, showed only a small and not significant change. This can also be seen from Fig. 3, where these data are presented in the form of a graph.

Table 2. Coronary haemodynamics and myocardial O_2 consumption after etomidate (same investigation). MBF = myocardial blood flow, CVR = coronary vascular resistance, MDAP = mean diastolic arterial pressure (coronary perfusion pressure), $M\dot{V}O_2$ = myocardial O_2 consumption, O_2Sat. cor.-ven. = O_2-Sat. coronary sinus, $AVDO_2$ = arterio-coronary venous oxygen difference

		Control		Etomidate		Change (%)
		$\bar{x}$	$s_{\bar{x}}$	$\bar{x}$	$s_{\bar{x}}$	
MBF	(ml/min·100g)	88	4	105[a]	4	+ 19
CVR	($\frac{mm\ Hg}{ml/min·100g}$)	0.89	0.05	0.72[b]	0.03	- 19
MDAP	(mm Hg)	81	2	79	2	——
$M\dot{V}O_2$	(ml/min·100g)	10.5	0.8	11.1	0.8	——
O_2Sat cor-ven (%)		29.7	1	35.8[b]	1	+ 21
AVD-O_2	(Vol.-%)	11.8	0.6	10.5[b]	0.5	- 11

[a] $p < 0.025$;   [b] $p < 0.01$

Table 3. Cardiovascular effects of 1.5 μg/kg fentanyl and a following injection of 0.3 mg/kg etomidate for induction of anaesthesia in 10 patients with heart valve disease NYH-Ass. classification III-IV. Mean ($\bar{x}$) and S.E.M. ($s_{\bar{x}}$). SAP (systolic), DAP (diastolic), MAP (mean) arterial pressure, HR (heart rate), CI (cardiac index), SVI (stroke volume index), TPR (total peripheral resistance)

	Control		Fentanyl (1.5γ/kg)		Etomidate (0.3 mg/kg)		P
SAP (mm Hg)	126	± 4	110	± 7	104	± 6	< 0.0005
DAP (mm Hg)	72	± 4	65	± 6	65	± 4	< 0.05
MAP (mm Hg)	90	± 4	80	± 5	78	± 3	< 0.01
HR (1/min)	85	± 7	88	± 7	78	± 5	n.s.
CI (1/min · m^2)	2.85	± 0.37	2.7	± 0.5	2.73	± 0.39	n.s.
SVI (ml/m^2)	34.0	± 2.88	34.8	± 6.3	39	± 3.87	n.s.
TPR ($\frac{mm\ Hg}{ml/min · kg}$)	1.29	± 0.3	1.2	± 0.3	1.15	± 0.24	n.s.

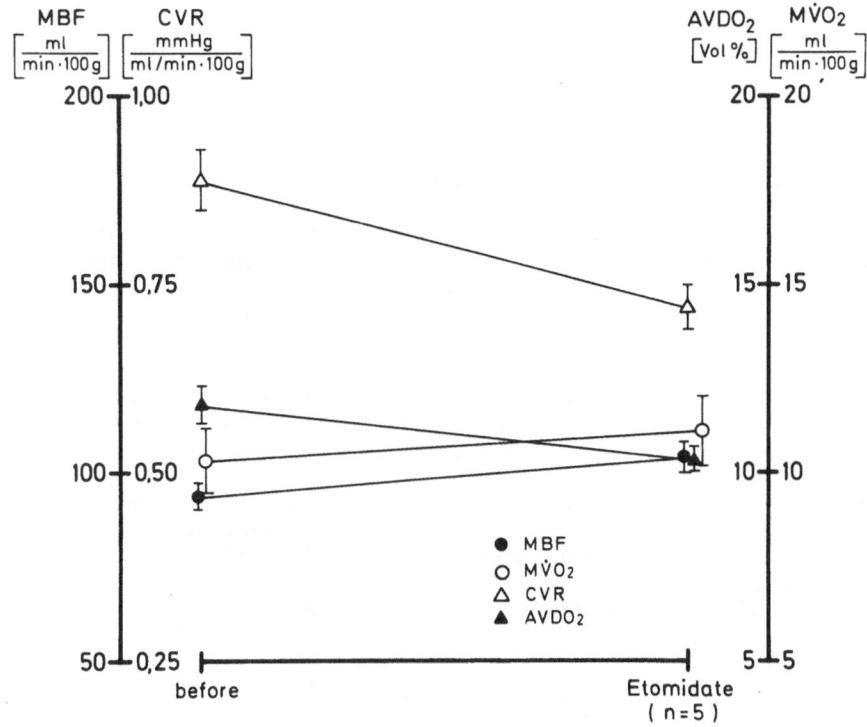

Fig. 3. *Illustration of the effect of 0.12 mg/kg · min etomidate on the coronary haemodynamics and M$\dot{V}O_2$ in a 35 year old female patient. Etomidate causes a mild increase in the myocardial blood flow (MBF) and a corresponding decrease in the coronary vascular resistance (CVR). Because of a simultaneous decrease in the arterio-coronary venous O_2 difference (AVDO$_2$), the myocardial O_2 consumption (M$\dot{V}O_2$) remains practically unchanged*

Second Part of the Study

In this group of patients with known heart valve disease the systolic arterial pressure (SAP) decreased by 17 % and MAP by 13 %. Heart rate, CI, SVI and TRP were not influenced significantly. (Table 3)

Discussion

Our group of investigators has recently reported on the importance of haemodynamic changes under conditions of anaesthesia with respect to the oxygen supply of the myocardium (7). Decisive haemodynamic determinants for the myocardial O_2 requirement are the contractility and the systolic wall tension of the left ventricle and the heart rate (9). Since both the preload (left ventricular enddiastolic pressure) and the afterload (aortic pressure) remain the same under the action of etomidate, the fact that the values of dp/dt$_{max}$ also show no significant change may

be interpreted as indicating an unimpaired function of the heart.

The slight increase in the heart rate (81/min to 88/min) did not lead to an increase in dp/dt_{max} in this low frequency range.

The systolic wall tension of the left ventricle, like the contractility and ventricular pressures, should also change only slightly. It appears from the above that the only possible cause of an increase in the O_2 consumption of the heart is the very small increase in the heart rate. However, the slight mean increase in the myocardial O_2 consumption under etomidate as compared to control values is not significant. Since the contractility and the stroke volume are not affected, the heart rate increase can best be explained by adaptation of the heart to a direct peripheral vasodilatory action of etomidate. The overall result is a moderate increase in the cardiac index. The observed decrease in the coronary resistance also points to a direct vascular action of etomidate. The increased coronary flow was balanced out by a simultaneous decrease in the coronary O_2 extraction, with the result that the oxygen uptake remained practically the same.

Good agreement therefore exists between the haemodynamic state and the energy consumption of the heart under the action of etomidate. Comparison of the cardiovascular effects of etomidate with those of other intravenous anaesthetics shows that etomidate offers definite haemodynamic advantages (Tables 4 and 5):

Table 4. Effects of various intravenous anaesthetics on mean arterial pressure (MAP), heart rate (HR) and maximal rate of left ventricular pressure rise (dp/dt_{max}) in a total of 60 patients without circulatory disease. Fentanyl was given after droperidol to complete neuroleptanalgesia (NLA). Mean ($\bar{x}$) and S.E.M. ($s_{\bar{x}}$)

	n	MAP (mm Hg) before	MAP (mm Hg) during	HR (b/min) before	HR (b/min) during	dp/dt_{max} (mm Hg/sec) before	dp/dt_{max} (mm Hg/sec) during
Ketamine	14	99+3	110+4 [3]	79+4	107+7 [4]	2050+68	2320+179
Droperidol +	10	105+4	91+4	77+3	94+4 [1]	2260+56	2370+ 54 [1]
Fentanyl (NLA)			93+4		79+3 [1]		2140+ 67 [1]
Methohexital	7	98+4	96+5	82+3	107+3 [4]	2030+98	1170+109 [3]
Thiopental	7	94+1	87+2 [3]	81+4	107+6 [3]	1280+59	1107+ 38 [3]
Etomidate	5	92+2	90+2	81+4	88+4 [2]	1160+49	1180+ 38
Propanidid	7	92+3	88+2 [1]	79+3	129+3 [4]	1510+89	1300+ 82 [1]
Althesin	7	97+4	91+3 [1]	79+4	114+9 [3]	1400+81	1470+ 79 [1]
Cremophor EL	3	92+2	90+2	80+2	78+5	1490+76	1440+ 48

1) p<0.05; 2) p<0.01; 3) p<0.0025; 4) p<0.0005

Table 5. Effects of various intravenous anaesthetics on cardiac index (CI), stroke volume index (SVI) and total peripheral resistance (TPR) in a total of 60 patients. Mean ($\bar{x}$) and S.E.M. ($s_{\bar{x}}$)

	n	CI ($l/min \cdot m^2$) before	CI during	SVI (ml/m^2) before	SVI during	TPR ($\frac{mm\ Hg}{ml/min \cdot kg}$) before	TPR during
Ketamine	14	3.77 ± 0.13	3.68 ± 0.23	49 ± 2	37 ± 3[2]	0.99 ± 0.06	1.21 ± 0.10[2]
Droperidol +	10	3.72 ± 0.09	3.93 ± 0.09	48 ± 2	45 ± 2	0.99 ± 0.05	0.84 ± 0.05[3]
Fentanyl (NLA)			3.43 ± 0.10		44 ± 3		0.98 ± 0.08[3]
Methohexital	7	3.99 ± 0.14	3.75 ± 0.17	50 ± 4	35 ± 2[2]	0.97 ± 0.07	0.99 ± 0.10
Thiopental	7	3.80 ± 0.21	3.20 ± 0.25[3]	48 ± 3	31 ± 4[3]	0.96 ± 0.07	1.05 ± 0.09
Etomidate	5	3.44 ± 0.17	3.93 ± 0.15[2]	43 ± 3	45 ± 4	1.05 ± 0.11	0.92 ± 0.09[2]
Propanidid	7	3.91 ± 0.11	3.63 ± 0.19[1]	47 ± 2	30 ± 2[3]	1.01 ± 0.05	0.93 ± 0.06[3]
Althesin	7	3.44 ± 0.08	4.17 ± 0.41[3]	43 ± 1 8	37 ± 3 5[1]	1.01 ± 0.09	0.84 ± 0.07[2]
Cremophor EL	3	3.87 ± 0.20	3.90 ± 0.24	46 ± 2	46 ± 1	1.01 ± 0.04	0.96 ± 0.6

1) $p < 0.05$; 2) $p < 0.01$; 3) $p < 0.0025$

Table 6. Effects of various intravenous anaesthetics on myocardial blood flow (MBF), myocardial oxygen consumption ($\dot{M}VO_2$), arterio-coronary venous O_2 difference ($AVDO_2$) and coronary vascular resistance (CVR) in a total of 60 patients. Mean ($\bar{x}$) and S.E.M. ($s_{\bar{x}}$).

	n	MBF (ml/min x 100 g)		$\dot{M}VO_2$ (ml/min x 100 g)		$AVDO_2$ (Vol. %)		CVR ($\frac{mm\ Hg}{ml/min\ x\ 100\ g}$)	
Ketamine	14	92 ± 5	168 ± 21[3]	11.1 ± 0.6	18.4 ± 2.0[3]	11.9 ± 0.3	11.9 ± 0.4	0.94 ± 0.04	0.66 ± 0.07[3]
Droperidol +	10	97 ± 7	139 ± 13[2]	10.3 ± 0.8	14.3 ± 1.0[2]	10.8 ± 0.6	10.9 ± 0.7	0.91 ± 0.06	0.60 ± 0.03[3]
Fentanyl (NLA)			92 ± 7[2]		9.2 ± 0.5[2]		10.4 ± 0.7		0.93 ± 0.07[3]
Methohexital	7	93 ± 3	126 ± 6[3]	10.9 ± 0.6	15.1 ± 1.1[3]	10.8 ± 0.4	11.9 ± 0.5	0.90 ± 0.07	0.65 ± 0.05[3]
Thiopental	7	83 ± 4	129 ± 8[3]	9.2 ± 0.6	14.3 ± 0.8[3]	10.9 ± 0.4	11.1 ± 0.5	0.97 ± 0.05	0.62 ± 0.06[3]
Etomidate	5	88 ± 4	105 ± 4[2]	10.5 ± 0.8	11.1 ± 0.8	11.8 ± 0.6	10.5 ± 0.5[2]	0.89 ± 0.05	0.72 ± 0.03[1]
Propanidid	7	93 ± 4	182 ± 10[3]	10.6 ± 0.6	19.3 ± 1.6[3]	11.4 ± 0.4	11.1 ± 0.6	0.92 ± 0.04	0.43 ± 0.03[3]
Althesin	7	96 ± 2	173 ± 22[3]	10.8 ± 0.9	18.6 ± 2.7[3]	11.1 ± 0.8	11.0 ± 0.9	0.90 ± 0.01	0.52 ± 0.06[3]
Cremophor EL	3	92 ± 4	97 ± 9	10.5 ± 0.5	10.8 ± 1.9	11.2 ± 0.5	11.1 ± 0.9	0.90 ± 0.05	0.84 ± 0.09

1) $p < 0.05$; 2) $p < 0.01$; 3) $p < 0.005$

1. It has less effect on the heart rate than propanidid, ketamine, Althesin, and the barbiturates. With regard to the comparable values under complete NLA, it must be remembered that droperidol alone leads to a considerable increase in the heart rate, which is balanced out by fentanyl (6, 7).

2. Etomidate does not lead either to a decrease (propanidid, Althesin) or to an (often undesirable) increase (ketamine) in the aortic pressure. Similar favourable behaviour is observed with methohexital and thiopental.

3. All the other anaesthetics investigated, with the exception of NLA, caused a decrease in the stroke volume, which was partly offset by the increase in the heart rate. With etomidate, on the other hand, the stroke volume is unchanged, and the cardiac index increases slightly.

4. Etomidate exhibits similar advantages with regard to inotropic behaviour, as measured by the dp/dt_{max}, which is neither negatively nor positively affected by this agent.

5. Unlike ketamine and like propanidid and Althesin etomidate leads to a slight decrease in the peripheral vascular resistance. This comparison also favours etomidate with respect to the energy loading of the heart (Table 6). With the exception of complete NLA (droperidol alone leads to a strong increase) all the other preparations compared cause a more or less pronounced increase in the oxygen consumption of the myocardium. As with the other anaesthetics, an increase in the coronary blood flow is observed. in the case of etomidate. However, this is not due to an increased O_2 requirement, but may be regarded as resulting from a weak true coronary dilatory effect of etomidate, which would appear to be of no further clinical consequence.

Also in the second part of the study, in which induction of anaesthesia in 10 patients with heart valve disease was performed, only small changes of the haemodynamics were observed. It should be noted, however, that arterial pressure drop is more pronounced and occurs already after the proceeding fentanyl injection (Table 3).

It was of particular interest that a premedication consisting of droperidol, fentanyl and atropine, and an additional injection of 1.5 μg/kg fentanyl i.v. prior to etomidate was able to offset the neurological side effects found in part one of this study.

If one considers the cardiovascular effects by themselves, etomidate is found to offer considerable advantages over the other intravenous anaesthesia methods investigated. The induction of anaesthesia with etomidate could be particularly advantageous for patients with reduced cardiovascular function, shock patients, and coronary risk patients.

It should be emphasized that etomidate is best used in clinical practice in combination with a potent neuroleptic and analgetic premedication.

92

Summary

The effects of the new intravenous hypnotic agent etomidate
(0.12 mg/kg · min) on the general and coronary haemodynamics,
myocardial blood flow (MBF) and myocardial oxygen consumption
($M\dot{V}O_2$) were studied on 5 unpremedicated patients undergoing
thoracic or vascular surgery. In a second part of the study general haemodynamics were analyzed before and after induction of
anaesthesia with 0.3 mg/kg etomidate in 10 patients scheduled
for heart valve replacement. This group of patients received a
premedication of 5 mg droperidol, 0.1 mg fentanyl and 0.5 mg
atropine. In addition 1.5 μg/kg fentanyl i.v. was given prior
to application of etomidate. In both groups general haemodynamics
changed only slightly and were more pronounced in the patients
with heart valve disease.
Accordingly, $M\dot{V}O_2$ remained unchanged, accompanied by a small
increase of MBF. There was a corresponding decrease in the coronary oxygen extraction.
Compared with the other intravenous anaesthetics Althesin, ketamine, methohexital, propanidid, thiopental, and droperidol (part
of neuroleptanalgesia) etomidate appeared to produce only small
effects on the haemodynamics and less increase in MBF and $M\dot{V}O_2$.
Therefore, etomidate might be advantageous for induction of
anaesthesia in cardiovascular risk patients, particularly when
the coronary reserve is reduced.
Because of certain undesirable side effects, particularly myocloni, and absence of an analgesic property, etomidate should be
used in combination with a potent neuroleptic and/or analgesic
agent, such as droperidol and fentanyl.

Zusammenfassung

An 5 nicht prämedizierten kreislaufgesunden Patienten wurden im
Rahmen einer Narkoseeinleitung die Herz-Kreislaufwirkungen ein-
schließlich der coronaren Hämodynamik und des myokardialen Sauerstoffverbrauchs des neuen intravenösen Hypnotikums Etomidate
(0,12 mg/kg KG min) untersucht.
In einem zweiten Teil der Studie wurden die allgemeinen Kreislauf
reaktionen vor und nach Narkoseeinleitung mit 0,3 mg/kg Etomidate
an 10 Patienten mit Herzklappenfehlern (New York-Heart-Association
Klassifikation III-IV), die sich einer Herzklappenersatzoperation
unterziehen mußten, gemessen. Diese Patientengruppe erhielt vor
der Etomidate-Injektion eine Prämedikation von 5 mg Dehydrobenzperidol und 0,1 mg Fentanyl sowie 0,5 mg Atropin. Zusätzlich
wurde unmittelbar vor der Applikation von Etomidate 1,5 μg/kg
Fentanyl intravenös gegeben. In beiden Gruppen kam es nur zu
geringen Veränderungen der gemessenen hämodynamischen Parameter.
Diese Veränderungen waren jedoch in der Patientengruppe mit Klap-
penfehlern stärker betont. Entsprechend den hämodynamischen
Veränderungen blieb der myokardiale Sauerstoffverbrauch trotz
einer geringfügigen Zunahme der Coronardurchblutung unverändert,
da die arterio-coronarvenöse Sauerstoffdifferenz abnahm. Vergli-
chen mit anderen intravenösen Anaesthetika (Althesin, Ketamine,
Methohexital, Propanidid, Thiopental und Dehydrobenzperidol)
fanden sich nach Etomidate wesentlich geringere Veränderungen

der hämodynamischen Parameter, der Myokarddurchblutung und des myokardialen Sauerstoffverbrauchs. Aufgrund unserer Untersuchungen schließen wir, daß Etomidate für die Narkoseeinleitung bei kardiovaskulären Risikopatienten, insbesondere bei reduzierter Coronarreserve, gut geeignet ist. Wegen einiger unerwünschter Nebenwirkungen (Myoklonie, Fehlen jeglicher analgetischer Eigenschaft) sollte Etomidate stets in Kombination mit einer ausreichenden Prämedikation und während der Narkoseeinleitung in Verbindung mit einem starken analgetischen Pharmakon wie Fentanyl verwendet werden.

References

1. BRETSCHNEIDER, H.J., COTT, L.A., HENSEL, I., KETTLER, D., MARTEL, J.: Ein neuer komplexer hämodynamischer Parameter aus 5 additiven Gliedern zur Bestimmung des O_2-Bedarfs des linken Ventrikels. Pflügers Arch. ges. Physiol. 319, R 14 (1970).

2. BRÜCKNER, J.B., GETHMANN, J.W., PATSCHKE, D., TARNOW, J., WEYMAR, A.: Untersuchungen zur Wirkung von Etomidate auf den Kreislauf des Menschen. Anaesthesist 23, 322 (1974).

3. DOENICKE, A.: Klinisch-experimentelle Untersuchungen und erster klinischer Erfahrungsbericht über ein neues i.v. Hypnoticum. Proceedings: 6. Internationaler Fortbildungskurs für klinische Anaesthesiologie, Wien, 21.-25. Mai 1973.

4. DOENICKE, A., GABANYI, D., LEMEE, H., SCHÜRK-BULICH, M.: Kreislaufverhalten und Myokardfunktion nach drei kurzwirkenden i.v. Hypnotica: Etomidate, Propanidid, Methohexital. Anaesthesist 23, 108 (1974).

5. DOENICKE, A., WAGNER, E., BEETZ, K.H.: Blutgasanalysen (arteriell) nach drei kurzwirkenden i.v. Hypnotica (Propanidid, Etomidate, Methohexital). Anaesthesist 22, 353 (1973).

6. JANSSEN, P.A.J., NIEMEGEERS, C.J.E., SCHELLEKENS, K.H.L., LENAERTS, F.M.: Etomidate, R-(+)-Ethyl-1-(-methyl-benzyl) imidazole-5-carboxylate (R 16 659). Arzneimittel-Forsch. 21, 1234 (1971).

7. KETTLER, D.: Sauerstoffbedarf und Sauerstoffversorgung des Herzens in Narkose. Anaesthesiologie und Wiederbelebung, B. 67. Berlin-Heidelberg-New York: Springer 1973.

8. KETTLER, D., SONNTAG, H., DONATH, U., REGENSBURGER, D., SCHENK, H.-D.: Hämodynamik, Myokardmechanik, Sauerstoffbedarf und Sauerstoffversorgung des menschlichen Herzens unter Narkoseeinleitung mit Etomidate. Anaesthesist 23, 116 (1974).

9. SONNENBLICK, E.H.: The determinants of O_2-consumption of the heart. In: Reindell, H., Keul, J., Doll, E. (Hrsg.): Herzinsuffizienz, S. 271, Stuttgart 1968.

10. SONNTAG, H.: Coronardurchblutung und Energieumsatz des menschlichen Herzens unter verschiedenen Anaesthetica. Anaesthesiologie und Wiederbelebung, B. 79. Berlin-Heidelberg-New York: Springer 1973.

94

11. SONNTAG, H., HEISS, H.W., KNOLL, D., REGENSBURGER, D., SCHENK, H.-D.,
     BRETSCHNEIDER, H.-J.: Über die Myokarddurchblutung und den myokardialen
     Sauerstoffverbrauch bei Patienten während Narkoseeinleitung mit Dehydro-
     benzperidol/Fentanyl oder Ketamine. Z. Kreisl.-Forsch. 61, 1092 (1972).

12. SONNTAG, H., SCHENK, H.-D., KETTLER, D., HELLBERG, K., KNOLL, D.,
     DONATH, U., BECKER, H.: Effects of Althesin (CT 1341) on Coronary Blood
     Flow and Myocardial Metabolism in Man. Acta anaesth. scand. 17, 218
     (1973).

13. SONNTAG, H., HELLBERG, K., SCHENK, H.-D., DONATH, U., REGENSBURGER, D.,
     KETTLER, D., DUCHANOVA, H., LARSEN, R., KOTSERONIS, J.: Effects of
     Thiopental (Trapanal) on Coronary Blood Flow and Myocardial Metabolism
     in Man. Acta anaesth. scand. 19, 69 (1975).

14. SONNTAG, H., KETTLER, D., HEISS, H.W., TAUCHERT, M., REGENSBURGER, D.,
     PASCHEN, K., BRETSCHNEIDER, H.J.: Coronardurchblutung und myokardialer
     Sauerstoffverbrauch bei Patienten unter Ketamin. In: Anaesthesiologie
     und Wiederbelebung Bd. 80, S. 263. Berlin-Heidelberg-New York: Springer
     1974.

15. SCHENK, H.-D., SONNTAG, H., KETTLER, D., REGENSBURGER, D., DONATH, U.,
     KOTSERONIS, J., BRETSCHNEIDER, H.-J.: Der Einfluß von Epontol auf den
     Sauerstoffverbrauch des Herzens und die Hämodynamik beim Menschen.
     Anaesthesist 23, 105 (1974).

16. WEYMAR, A., EIGENHEER, F., GETHMANN, J.W., REINECKE, A., PATSCHKE, D.,
     TARNOW, J., BRÜCKNER, J.B.: Tierexperimentelle Untersuchungen zur Wir-
     kung von Etomidate (R 26 490-Sulfat) auf den Kreislauf und die myokardiale
     Sauerstoffversorgung. Anaesthesist 23, 150 (1974).

Experimental Investigations on the Direct Effect of Etomidate on Myocardial Contractility[+]

K.-J. Fischer and H. Marquort

The short-acting intravenous narcotics, such as propanidid, methohexital, ketamine and Althesin, developed in recent years, are not
devoid of undesirable cardiovascular side-effects (FISCHER, 1971,
1972, 1973; JAGENEAU et al., 1973; DOENICKE et al., 1974; KETTLER
et al., 1974 b; WEYMAR et al., 1974).

In search for compounds inducing a lower degree of cardiovascular
impairment, etomidate was synthetized (JANSSEN et al., 1971).
It appeared from animal experiments (JAGENEAU et al., 1973; WEYMAR
et al., 1974; FISCHER, MARQUORT, 1974), as well as from clinical
studies (DOENICKE et al., 1974; KETTLER et al., 1974 b; BRÜCKNER
et al., 1974; BRUGMANS et al., 1974; HEMPELMANN et al., 1974),
that the cardiovascular depressor effect of this short-acting
hypnotic is extremely low by comparison.

It was, therefore, of interest to directly examine the inotropic
and chronotropic effect of etomidate in the isolated heart. The
experiments were carried out in a modified heart-lung preparation
(PATTERSON, STARLING, 1914; KRAYER, 1931; FISCHER, 1971, 1972,
1973; BÖTTCHER et al., 1974). Thus, the myocardial function can
be studied without any interference by nerval or humoral influences (MASON, 1968; FISCHER, 1971, 1972, 1973; FISCHER, MARQUORT,
1974).

Changes of the heart rate, of the preload and afterload may interfere with the quantification of the myocardial contractility
modified by drugs. These parameters can, however, be kept constant
or can be controlled in the heart-lung preparation (MASON, 1968;
FISCHER, 1972, 1973; BÖTTCHER et al., 1974). This is warranted
by atrial stimulation at a constant rate, a fixed reservoir-blood
level and a constant "Starling-resistance".

Material and Methods

Heart-lung preparations were obtained from 24 cats of either sex
(mean b.w. 2.54 kg) under light chloralose anaesthesia (50 mg/kg
b.w., i.p.). The circulating blood volume amounted to 250 ml.
The temperature was kept constant at 37°C.

[+] Supported by Grant No. LU 31/17 from Deutsche Forschungsgemeinschaft

The following parameters were recorded on two 4-channel recording devices (HE 18, Hellige, Freiburg): ECG, aortic blood flow (electromagnetic flowmeter, Liepelt, Ahrensburg), aortic pressure, right ventricular and right atrial pressure (Statham model P 23 Db) and left ventricular pressure (micro-catheter tip manometer PC 350 A, Millar Instr., Houston/Texas). The maximum rate of left ventricular pressure rise (dp/dt_{max}) was differentiated via a RC-segment. To determine the contractile state of the beating heart, the maximum velocity of shortening (V_{max}) and the maximum measurable velocity of shortening ($V_{CE\ max}$) were obtained. The model for cardiac muscle used in the calculation of force-velocity relationship was that proposed by HILL (1938). This concept evaluated for skeletal muscle is applicable to the contractile mechanism of heart muscle, as SONNENBLICK (1962 a) has previously pointed out. Isovolemic contractions of the intact heart are equivalent to the isometric contractions of isolated heart muscle preparations. The isovolemic force-velocity curve was constructed by plotting V_{CE}, i.e. $(dp/dt)/32 \cdot IP)$, versus the instantaneously developed left ventricular pressure (I P). The factor 32 is a constant for the extensibility of the series elastic component and was adopted from investigations on isolated papillary heart muscle (MASON et al., 1971). As the velocity of shortening probably never reaches a maximum value in the intact heart because of the early onset of isotonic shortening, the theoretical velocity of shortening of the unloaded contractile element (V_{max}) can be approximated by extrapolating the isovolemic segment of the directly measured force-velocity curve to zero pressure load (SONNENBLICK 1962 a, 1962 b; MASON et al., 1969, 1971; SHIMOSATO, 1969; HUGENHOLTZ et al., 1970).

In order to assure comparable baseline conditions, the venous supply (constant reservoir-blood level, venous inflow = 25 ml/ kg b.w.), the peripheral pressure load ("STARLING-resistance" = 100 mm Hg) and the heart rate (atrial stimulation under constant rate) were kept constant. The rate of stimulation was set at 5 - 10 beats/min above the spontaneous heart rate. The impulse duration amounted to 0.5 m sec and the amplitude to 10 - 15 volts. Etomidate and hexobarbital were administered cumulatively into the venous reservoir. All measurements were done under steady state conditions.

In a second experimental series, the myocardial force was reduced by defined concentrations of the narcotic drugs, beginning with blood concentrations of hexobarbital which reduced dp/dt_{max} by 10, 25, 50, and 75 %, resp. (ED_{10}, ED_{25}, ED_{50}, ED_{75}). The results thus obtained were compaired with equinarcotic concentrations of etomidate.

The etomidate solvent (a 60 % aqueous propylene glycol solution) did not cause any change in contractility, even in concentrations up to 10 ml / 100 ml BV (blood volume) (FISCHER, MARQUORT, 1974).

Results

At first the concentration-response curves were established for
both hexobarbital and etomidate (Fig. 1). The effect was expressed
as percentage decrease of dp/dt_{max}. The influence of the two
substances was similar in quality: in the case of etomidate, the
ED_{25} was found to be 3.66 mg/100 ml BV, and the ED_{50} 6.52 mg/
100 ml BV. The corresponding values for hexobarbital amounted
to 9.0 and 17.5 mg/100 ml BV.
With respect to the therapeutic index, the relative distance
between the minimum narcotic concentration (ED_N) and the cardio-
depressive concentration (ED_{25} and ED_{50}, respectively) is of
particular interest.

In the case of etomidate (ED_N 0.47 mg/kg b.w. versus 3.66 and
6.52 mg/100 ml BV) a considerably larger therapeutic range
results as compared with hexobarbital (ED_N 5.6 mg/kg b.w. versus
9.0 and 17.5 mg/100 ml BV) (FISCHER, MARQUORT, 1974).

Fig. 2 summarizes the changes of the haemodynamic parameters
related to the corresponding equinarcotic concentrations of
hexobarbital and etomidate, respectively. The maximum rate of
left ventricular pressure rise (dp/dt_{max}) can be taken as an
indirect measure of the velocity of shortening of the contractile
elements under constant and controlled conditions (SONNENBLICK
1962 b; MITCHELL et al., 1963; BRAUNWALD et al., 1968; HERPFER,
1970; MORGENSTERN et al., 1972; BARNES et al., 1973; KÖHLER,
MESCHER, 1973).

With logarithmically increasing concentrations of hexobarbital,
dp/dt_{max} linearily decreased from 1796 to 469 mm Hg/sec between
ED_{10} and ED_{75}. In contrast the negative inotropic effect of
equinarcotic concentrations of etomidate (0.4 - 2.43 mg/100 ml
BV) was found to be small, dp/dt_{max} only being reduced from
1527 to 1208 mm Hg/sec. Within this concentration range the left
ventricular peak systolic pressure is comparable to the observed
decrease of dp/dt_{max}. As far as the stroke volume is concerned,
the two drugs acted similarly within the concentration ranges
investigated. With higher blood levels, however, the effect of
hexobarbital was somewhat more pronounced.

In contrast to the rather moderate influence of etomidate upon
the parameters mentioned (Table 1) the reduction of the aortic
stroke volume was the most striking result. Within the concentration range investigated the aortic stroke was reduced by 15.2,
24.3, 35.7, and 46.1 %, respectively, and by equinarcotic
concentrations of hexobarbital by 14.3, 27.1, 39.2, and 87.6 %,
respectively.

The estimation of the contractile state by means of the force-
velocity curves demonstrated a significantly smaller impairment
by etomidate than by equinarcotic concentrations of hexobarbital.

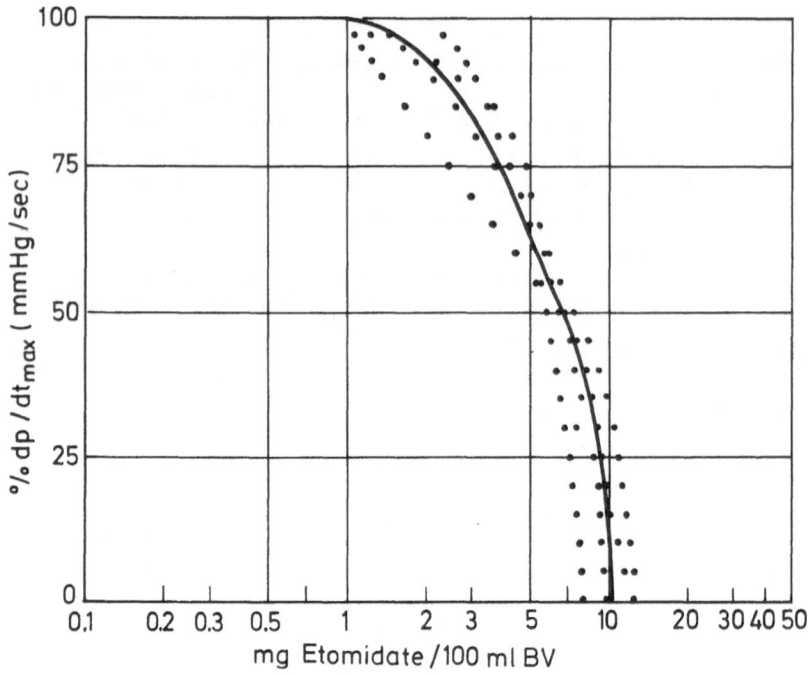

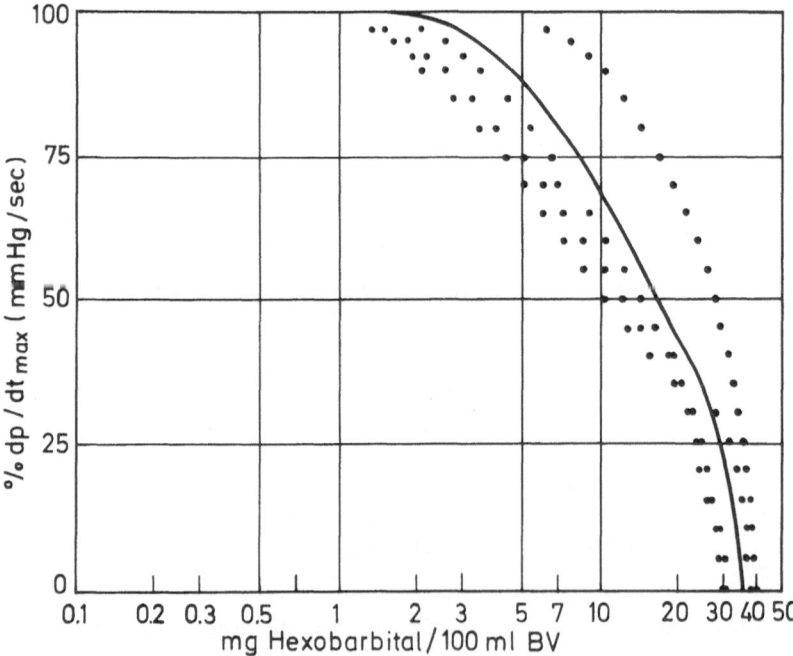

Fig. 1. Dose-response curves of etomidate and hexobarbital, respectively, in isolated electrically driven cat hearts (heart-lung preparation). Abscissa: concentration of the cumulatively administered narcotics. Ordinate: change of dp/dt_{max} in %

e 1. Changes in various cardiac parameters provoked by the highest inves-
ted etomidate concentration (2.43 mg/100 ml BV are equivalent to the ED_{50}
exobarbital): Aortic stroke volume (SV), maximum left ventricular pressure
(dp/dt$_{max}$), left ventricular peak systolic pressure (P_{LV}), mean diastolic
ic pressure (MAP$_{diast.}$), left ventricular enddiastolic pressure (LVEDP),
t ventricular peak systolic pressure (P_{RV}), right ventricular enddiastolic
sure (RVEDP), and heart rate (HR)

	Control	Etomidate 2.43 mg/100 ml BV	Δ %
ml)	0.375	0.291	− 41.6
It$_{max}$ Hg • sec^{-1})	1527	1208	− 20.9
(mm Hg)	108	103.7	− 4
liast. Hg)	87.6	80.8	− 7.8
)P (mm Hg)	4.5	10.4	+ 131.1
(mm Hg)	21.3	21.7	+ 1.9
)P (mm Hg)	2.9	4.8	+ 65.5
(1/min)	139.2	128.9	− 7.4

s holds true both for the measured ($V_{CE\ max}$) and for the
rapolated (V_{max}) maximum velocity of shortening of the contrac-
e elements (Fig. 3). The $V_{CE\ max}$ value of the controls was
2 ML/sec (muscle length/sec). At concentrations of hexo-
bital equal to ED_{50} (17.5 mg/100 ml BV) it was reduced to
ML/sec, and with equinarcotic concentrations of etomidate
y to 1,38 ML/sec. V_{max} of 2.81 ML/sec (controls) was diminished
1.26 ML/sec by hexobarbital but only 1.8 ML/sec by etomidate.

analogy to the FRANK-STARLING mechanism, the analysis of the
tricular function curves permits a qualitative evaluation of
force of contraction (SARNOFF, MITCHELL, 1962; GUYTON, 1968,
1; MORGENSTERN et al., 1972). An insufficient heart displays
urve which is flattened and shifted to the lower right,
licating a reduced cardiac output at identical right atrial
ling pressures (Fig. 4). A comparison of equinarcotic concen-
tions of hexobarbital and etomidate again demonstrates that
contractility was much less impaired by etomidate than by
obarbital (Fig. 5).

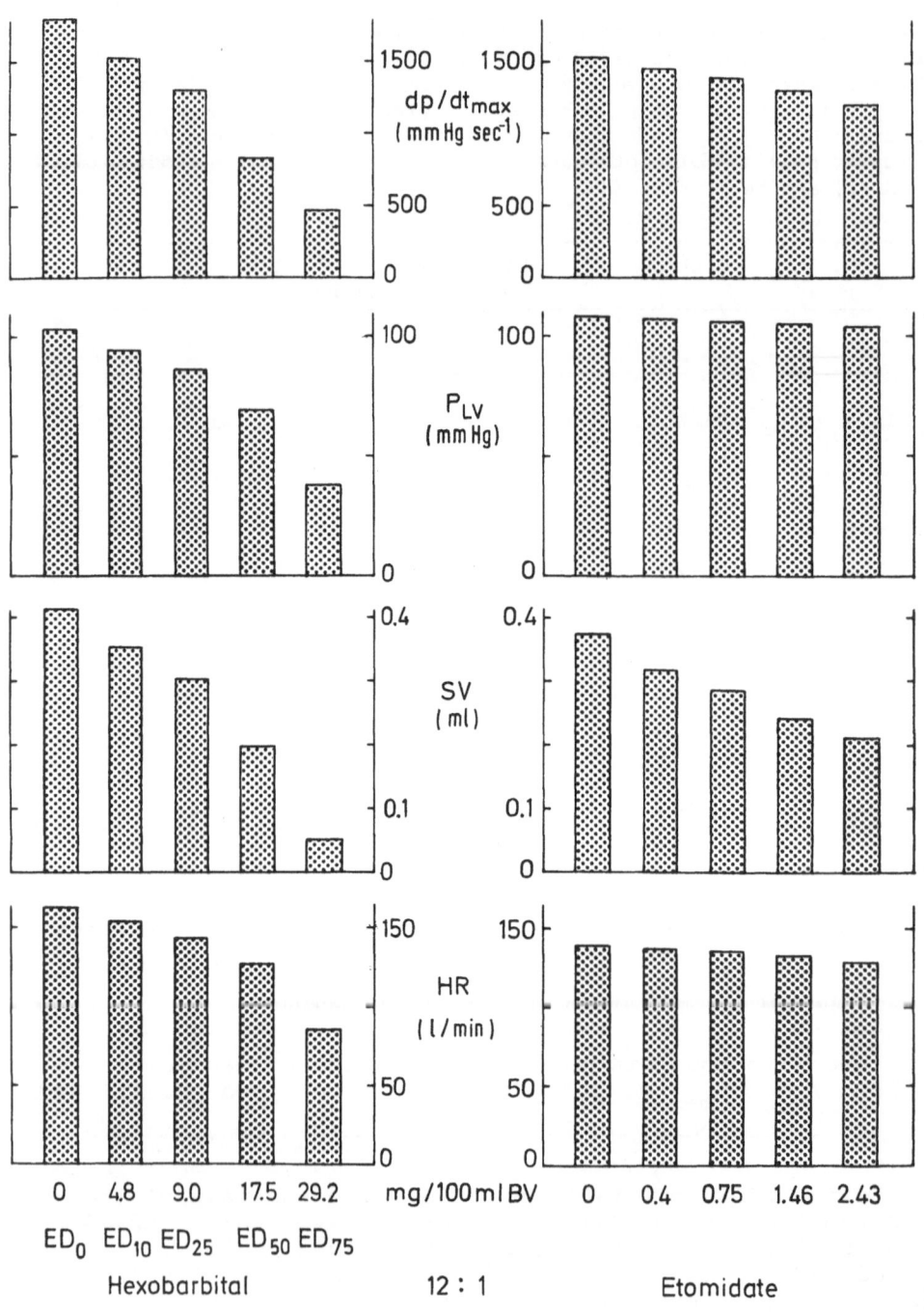

Fig. 2.Influence of equinarcotic concentrations of hexobarbital and etoï (12 : 1) on various cardiac parameters: maximum left ventricular pressu. rise (dp/dt$_{max}$), left ventricular peak systolic pressure (P$_{LV}$), aortic volume (SV), and spontaneous heart rate (HR)

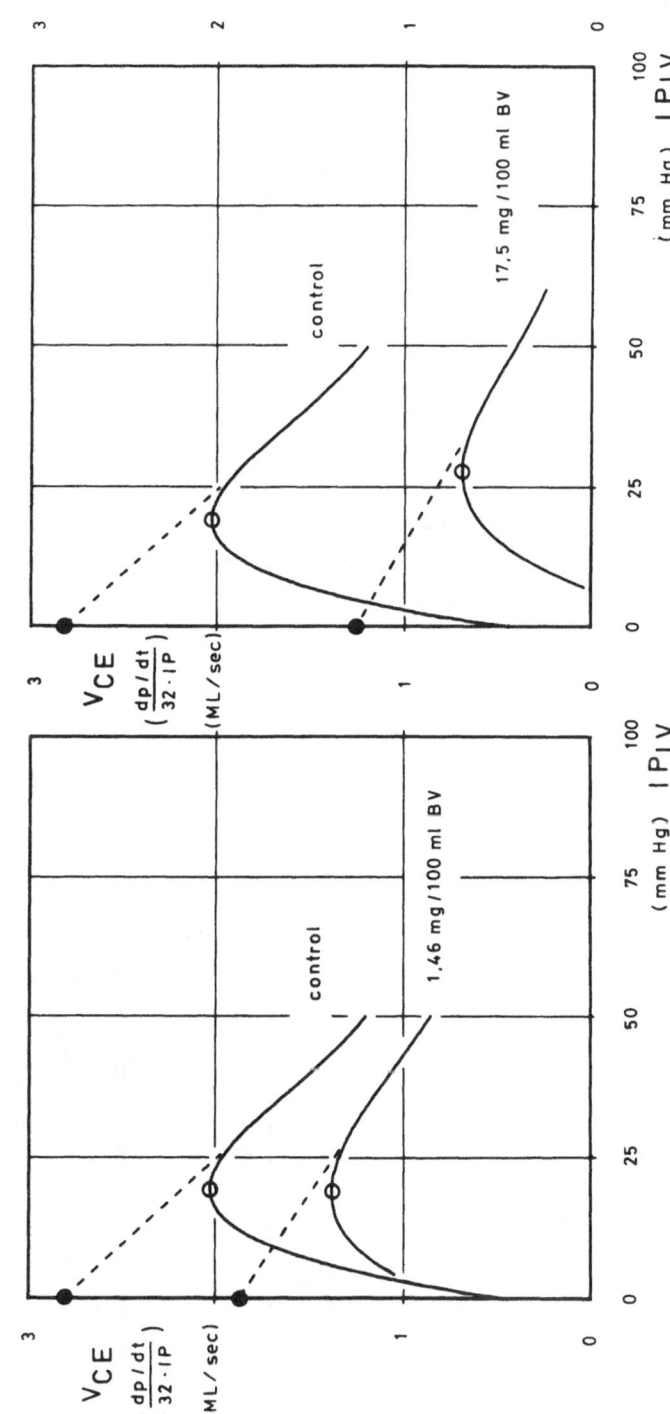

Fig. 3. Force-velocity curves (5th-order polynomials) determined at equinarcotic concentrations of etomidate and hexobarbital. V_{CE} (on the ordinate), $V_{CE\ max}$ (O) and V_{max} (●) are expressed as the relation $(dp/dt)/(32 \cdot IP)$ to instantaneously developed left ventricular pressure (IP_{LV}), where dp/dt is rate of isovolumetric left ventricular pressure rise and 32 is the series elastic constant. The broken lines represent the extrapolation of the isovolemic segment of the curve to V_{max} at zero load

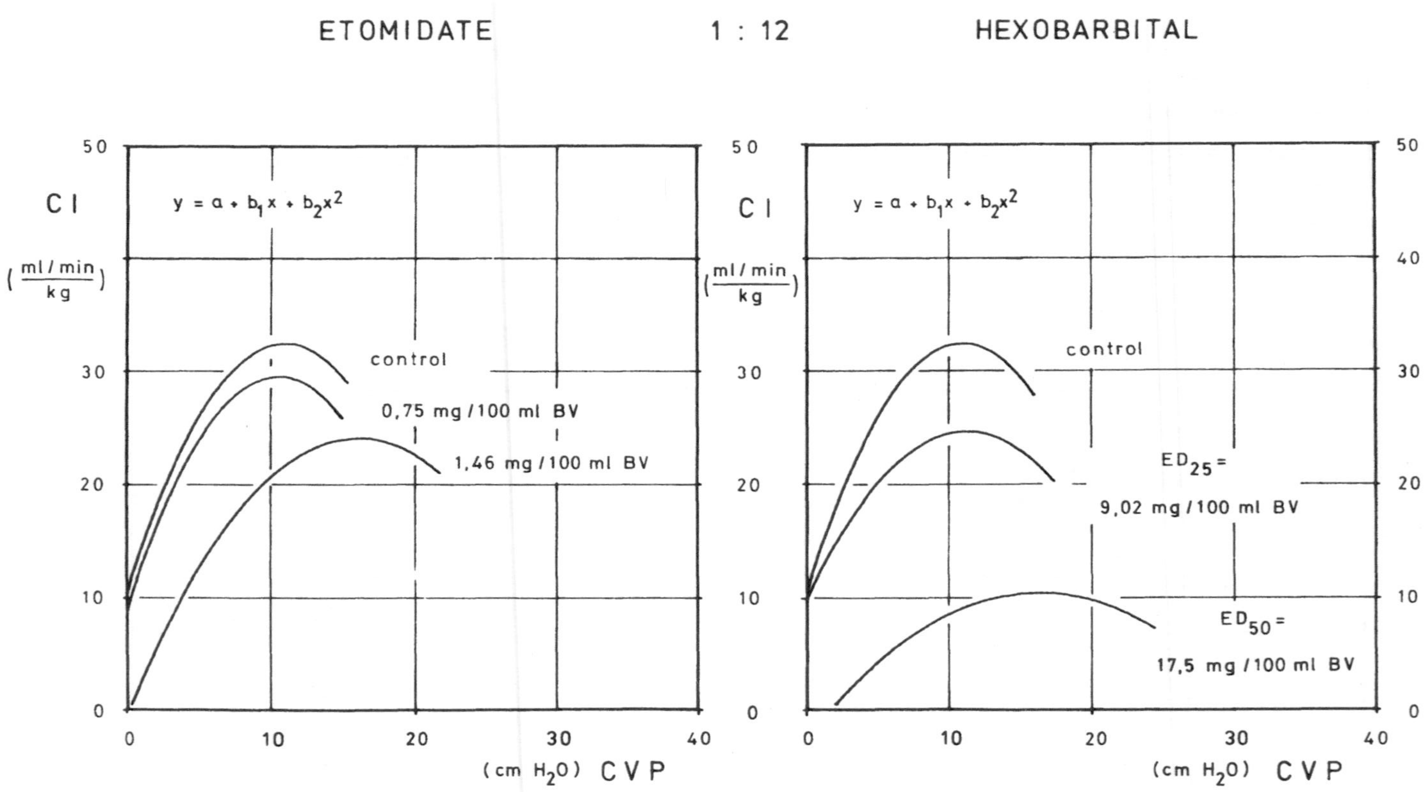

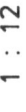

Fig. 4. *Ventricular function curves relating cardiac index (C I = aortic stroke volume/min • kg b.w.) to mean right atrial filling pressure (CVP). The regression curves (2nd-order polynomials) were obtained in controls and at equinarcotic concentrations of etomidate and hexobarbital*

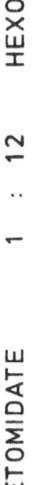

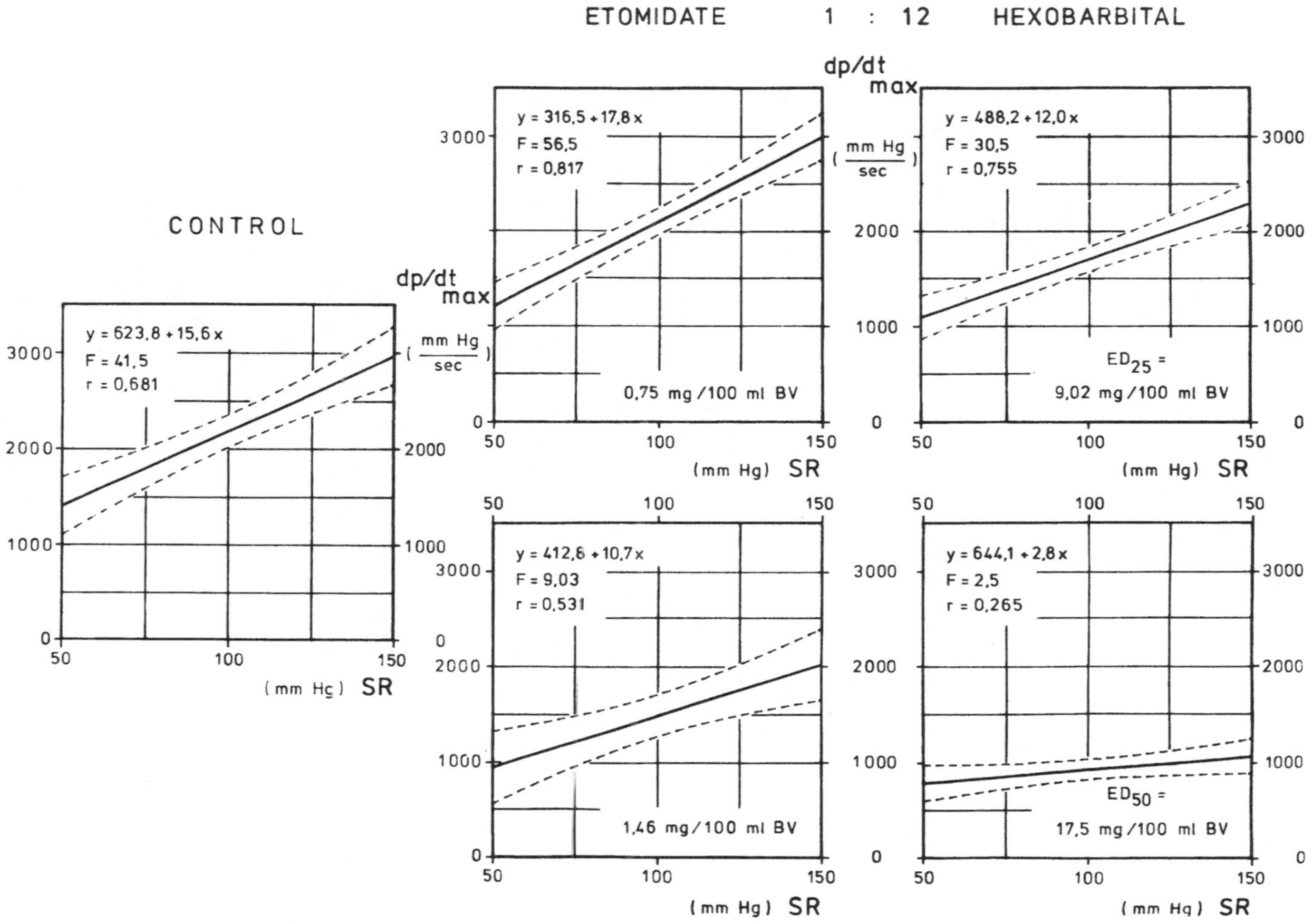
ETOMIDATE 1 : 12 HEXOBARBITAL
CONTROL
y = 623,8 + 15,6 x
F = 41,5
r = 0,681
y = 316,5 + 17,8 x
F = 56,5
r = 0,817
0,75 mg/100 ml BV
y = 488,2 + 12,0 x
F = 30,5
r = 0,755
ED25 =
9,02 mg/100 ml BV
y = 412,6 + 10,7 x
F = 9,03
r = 0,531
1,46 mg/100 ml BV
y = 644,1 + 2,8 x
F = 2,5
r = 0,265
ED50 =
17,5 mg/100 ml BV
dp/dt max
(mm Hg / sec)
(mm Hg) SR
0
1000
2000
3000
50
100
150

Fig. 5. Myocardial adaptability to defined pressure loads as determined by a gradual increase in "STARLING-resistance" (SR). Influence of equinarcotic concentrations of etomidate and hexobarbital. The linear regression curves (+ limits of 95 % confidence) are expressed as the relation of dp/dt_{max} *to the "STARLING-resistance"*

In the latter case, a right atrial filling pressure of 10 cm
H_2O resulted in a cardiac index (CI) of 24.5 and 8 ml/min · kg
b.w. for ED_{25} and ED_{50}, respectively. The corresponding values
for equivalent concentrations of etomidate were 29.0 and 21.5 ml/
min · kg b.w. The control value amounted to 32.5 ml/min · kg b.w.

The myocardial adaptability to altered afterloads can be studied
by a gradual increase of the "STARLING-resistance" from 50 -
100 mm Hg. In this range a linear correlation was found between
the increase of the "STARLING-resistance" and the increase of
mean diastolic aortic pressure (FISCHER, MARQUORT, 1974). The
augmentation of the afterload causes a significant increase of
the maximum rate of left ventricular pressure rise (NOBLE et al.,
1969; NOBLE, 1972; BRAUNWALD, 1972; STRAUER, 1973). In the case
of hexobarbital, already the ED_{25} reduced the cardiac response
to increasing afterloads, whereas the adaptation was completely
absent with concentrations equivalent to the ED_{50}. Following the
administration of etomidate, however, myocardial adaptation was
fully maintained at the lower concentration and only moderately
impaired at a concentration equivalent to the ED_{50} of hexobarbital.

Discussion

The direct myocardial effect of narcotic drugs can only be determined properly in isolated hearts (FISCHER, 1973). For this pur-
pose, the heart-lung preparation is very well suited since it
permits the control of the essential factors determining myocardial contractility (FISCHER, 1971, 1972, 1973; FISCHER, MARQUORT,
1974; BÖTTCHER et al., 1974). In such a model changes of dp/dt_{max},
of V_{max} or of $V_{CE\ max}$ can be taken as a true measure of inotropism
(BRAUNWALD et al., 1968; SHIMOSATO, 1969; FISCHER, 1971; BRAUN-
WALD, 1972; MORGENSTERN et al., 1972; STRAUER, 1973; KÖHLER, 1973;
KÖHLER, MESCHER, 1973; BARNES et al., 1973). The heart-lung preparation furthermore allows to apply defined changes of the pressure
and of the volume load and of the beating frequency (FISCHER,
MARQUORT, 1974).

A true comparison of direct myocardial effects of different
narcotics can be achieved if equinarcotic concentrations are
applied (FISCHER, 1973). In cats, the minimum hypnotic dosage
(ED_N) of hexobarbital was determined to be 5.59 mg/kg b.w. and
of etomidate 0.47 mg/kg b.w., resulting in an ED_N-ratio of 12 : 1
(FISCHER, MARQUORT, 1974). In cats, the hypnotic dosage of etomidate minimally exceeds that in man (0.15 - 0.3 mg/kg b.w.)
(DOENICKE et al., 1974; BRÜCKNER et al., 1974; BRUGMANS et al.,
1974; KETTLER et al, 1974 b; HEMPELMANN et al., 1974), but is
lower than in dogs (0.8 mg/kg b.w.) (JAGENEAU et al., 1973;
WEYMAR et al., 1974; TARNOW et al., 1974). At equinarcotic concentrations hexobarbital reduced the measured parameters to a greater
extent than etomidate.

No changes in spontaneous heart rate occured within the concentration range of 0.4 - 1.46 mg etomidate / 100 ml BV. Thus, the

direct negative inotropic effect preceeds the direct negative
chronotropic effect which is established at higher drug concentrations. Investigations in man (DOENICKE et al., 1974; KETTLER
et al., 1974 b; BRUGMANS et al., 1974; BRÜCKNER et al., 1974)
as well as experiments in intact animals (JAGENEAU et al., 1973;
WEYMAR et al., 1974) revealed a slight increase of the heart rate
in combination with other haemodynamic changes after the injection of a single hypnotic dose of etomidate. According to the
present observations, the increase in heart rate cannot be caused
by direct effects of etomidate upon the pacemaker. It might be
induced by a counter-regulation due to a peripheral vascular
dilation. HEMPELMANN et al. (1974), on the other hand, recorded
a fall of the heart rate by 11 % in patients with myocardial
damage.

In dogs, WEYMAR et al. (1974) observed a drop of aortic pressure
in combination with a marked augmentation of cardiac output and
an increase in heart rate. These findings can be explained as an
adaptation to the reduced total peripheral resistance. This
mechanism has been confirmed by investigations in man (BRÜCKNER
et al., 1974; KETTLER et al., 1974 b).

In the present study the most remarkable result was a severe
reduction of cardiac output (Fig. 2). At blood levels of 2.43 mg
etomidate / 100 ml BV, the aortic stroke volume decreased by
41.6 %. This cannot be the result of the diminished contractility
alone, as dp/dt_{max} is reduced by 20.9 % only. Furthermore, the
true reduction of contractility is a little higher as can be seen
in dp/dt_{max}-decrease: drop of mean diastolic aortic pressure by
7.8 % and increase in left ventricular enddiastolic pressure
by 5.9 mm Hg (Table 1) have to be taken into account (MORGENSTERN
et al., 1970; MASON, 1971; KÖHLER, 1973; STRAUER, 1973). Following
the administration of etomidate in man (0.12 mg/kg · min), a
decrease of the total peripheral and of the coronary vascular
resistance was calculated by Kettler et al. (1974 b). The corresponding increase of coronary blood flow amounted to 19 %, caused
by the dilating effect of etomidate. In the heart-lung preparation
peripheral systemic vascular resistance cannot change, unless the
"STARLING-resistance" is kept constant.
Provided that the specific coronary vascular site of action
(KETTLER et al., 1974 b) also applies to the cat heart muscle
preparations, the marked decrease of the stroke volume observed
in the present study might partly be explained as a result of a
disproportional increase of the coronary fraction of cardiac
output. Thus, the severe reduction of aortic stroke volume may
be caused by the decrease of contractile force and by a relative
increase in coronary stroke volume. In addition to these possibilities it cannot be decided if the influence of the direct
negative inotropic effect of etomidate is of the same extent
during the isometric, the isotonic, and the auxotonic phases of
the cardiac cycle.

The maximum rate of left ventricular pressure rise is considered
as a quantitative measure of contractility as long as the above
mentioned determinants (preload, afterload, frequency of

contraction) are kept constant or can be controlled (SONNENBLICK, 1962 b; MITCHELL et al., 1963; BRAUNWALD et al., 1968; HERPFER, 1970; MORGENSTERN et al., 1972; KÖHLER, 1973; BARNES et al., 1973). The decrease of dp/dt_{max} induced by etomidate is rather slight in contrast to a marked reduction by hexobarbital. Following the administration of 0.75 and 1.46 mg etomidate / 100 ml BV, dp/dt_{max} is reduced by 9.4 and 14.8 %, respectively, whereas the decrease by equipotent concentrations of hexobarbital (ED_{25} and ED_{50}) amounts to 27.5 and 53.8 %, respectively.

In intact animals (JAGENEAU et al., 1973; WEYMAR et al., 1974) and in man (KETTLER et al., 1974 b; BRÜCKNER et al., 1974; BRUG-MANS et al., 1974), the decrease of dp/dt_{max} by etomidate is extremely small. This becomes particularly evident in comparison with equinarcotic dosages of other short-acting intravenous narcotics (KETTLER et al., 1974 b; WEYMAR et al., 1974). However, these dp/dt_{max} values do not reflect the true changes in the inotropic state of the heart, as nerval and humoral influences can only be eliminated in isolated heart muscle preparations (FISCHER, 1971, 1972, 1973).

In evaluating the contractile state of the beating in situ heart, changes of the frequency of contraction, of preload and of after-load have to be taken into account (SONNENBLICK, 1962 a, 1962 b; MITCHELL et al., 1963; BRAUNWALD et al., 1968; MASON, 1968; NOBLE et al., 1969; MASON et al., 1969; MORGENSTERN et al., 1970; HERPFER, 1970; HUGENHOLTZ et al., 1970; MASON et al., 1971; MORGENSTERN et al., 1972; NOBLE, 1972; BRAUNWALD, 1972; MASON et al., 1972; KÖHLER, MESCHER, 1973; STRAUER, 1973; KÖHLER, 1973; BARNES et al., 1973; SCHMIDT et al., 1973; RAFF et al., 1974). This reserve also applies to the ratio dp/dt_{max}. In order to partly eliminate these falsifications, several contractility indices are in use (SIEGEL, SONNENBLICK, 1964; KRAYENBÜHL, 1969; MASON et al., 1971; FISCHER, 1971; BRAUNWALD, 1972; STRAUER, 1973; SCHMIDT et al., 1973; BARNES et al., 1973; RAFF et al., 1974).

The most reliable method available at present seems to be the quantification of myocardial inotropic state by means of the force-velocity relations (SONNENBLICK, 1962 a, 1962 b; SHIMOSATO, 1969; MASON et al., 1969; HUGENHOLTZ et al., 1970; MASON et al., 1971, 1972; STRAUER, 1973; SCHMIDT et al., 1973; KÖHLER, MESCHER, 1973). However, objections are raised, since extreme changes in preload particularly affect V_{max} values (NOBLE et al., 1969; NOBLE, 1972). Nevertheless, alterations in force-velocity relation have been shown to characterize the two general properties of heart muscle: a change in initial muscle length, which is the basis of the FRANK-STARLING mechanism, and a change in the contractile state of the heart as provoked by inotropic interventions (BRAUNWALD et al., 1968).

The decrease of contractility as determined by the force-velocity curves was found to be half of that determined for hexobarbital.

This becomes evident by the experimentally measured maximum velocity of shortening of the contractile elements ($V_{CE\,max}$), as well as by the extrapolated maximum velocity of shortening at a hypothetical zero load (V_{max}).

The results obtained with a single hypnotic dose of etomidate in intact animals (JAGENEAU et al., 1973; WEYMAR et al., 1974) and in man (DOENICKE et al., 1974; KETTLER et al., 1974 a, 1974 b; BRUGMANS et al., 1974; BRÜCKNER et al., 1974) suggest a rather moderate effect of etomidate on haemodynamics. The large therapeutic range of etomidate, compared to hexobarbital, can be explained by the relative distance between the ED_N and the ED_{25} or the ED_{50}. The concentrations of etomidate investigated (0,75 and 1.46 mg / 100 ml BV) lie still in the beginning portion of the dose-response curve. The equinarcotic concentrations of hexobarbital (9.0 and 17.5 mg / 100 ml BV), however, lie in the steep linear portion of the curve (Fig. 1). Thus, a marked reduction of contractility induced by etomidate cannot be expected in clinically relevant concentrations of this drug (FISCHER, MARQUORT, 1974).

The cardiovascular tolerance is narrowed under the influence of narcotics, especially in patients with a reduced coronary reserve, cardiac insufficiency, hypertension or in patients suffering from a decompensated haemorrhagic shock. This is also valid for etomidate: In patients with myocardial disease, HEMPELMANN et al., (1974) recorded a decrease of heart rate, dp/dt_{max}, left ventricular peak systolic pressure and cardiac index. A negative inotropic effect of etomidate in the case of previous myocardial insufficiency was also confirmed by KETTLER et al. (1974 a).

Ventricular function curves represent a qualitative measure of contractile force (SARNOFF, MITCHELL, 1962; GUYTON, 1968, 1971; MORGENSTERN et al., 1972; FISCHER, MARQUORT, 1974). The steepness of the curve within the range of normal right atrial filling pressures determines the degree of cardiac sufficiency. The slope of the curve beyond the peak is already an expression of cardiac decompensation.

The adaptation of cardiac performance to extreme volume loads is largely maintained in the presence of etomidate, but heavily reduced by equinarcotic concentrations of hexobarbital. An acute volume overload at concentrations of hexobarbital equivalent to the ED_{50} does not result in an adequate increase of cardiac output.

Alterations in the left ventricular afterload have a decisive effect on contractility parameters (MORGENSTERN et al., 1970, 1972; BRAUNWALD et al., 1972; STRAUER, 1973). In the case of constant heart rate and unchanged preload the sufficient heart shows a largely positive correlation between the increase of mean diastolic aortic pressure and the rise of dp/dt_{max}. With respect to the heart-lung preparation, the afterload can be increased separately by gradually augmenting the "STARLING-resistance". This allows the quantification of the adaptability of the intact heart to controlled alterations in afterload (FISCHER, MARQUORT, 1974). The cardiac capability to adapt is shown to be maintained under etomidate, even at higher blood concentrations of the drug. In contrast, the response to increasing afterload is missing in the presence of hexobarbital at equinarcotic concentrations.

Summary

In order to assess the qualitative and quantitative effects on myocardial contractile state induced by etomidate, dose-response correlations for this drug were established in the isolated, intact and beating heart (heart-lung preparation). There was only a slight direct negative inotropic effect at low and medium concentrations (< 1.5 mg/100 ml BV). A direct negative chronotropic effect was only detectable at higher drug concentrations. A comparison of equinarcotic concentrations of etomidate and hexobarbital revealed that etomidate possessed a significantly larger therapeutic range with regard both to inotropic and to chronotropic parameters. Nevertheless, a marked reduction of the aortic stroke volume by etomidate was noted, although all the other parameters remained rather constant. Testing the cardiac adaptability by gradual changes of volume and pressure loads at concentrations of etomidate or hexobarbital which caused a defined reduction of myocardial contractility, a much better ventricular performance was found in the presence of etomidate as compared to hexobarbital.
It may be concluded from the comparative study that etomidate might be advantageous as an induction hypnotic in patients with reduced cardiac reserve, since it only slightly depresses the myocardial contractility, and leaves the ventricular capability to adapt almost intact at narcotic concentrations.

Zusammenfassung

Die qualitativen und quantitativen Effekte von Etomidate auf den Kontraktilitätsstatus wurden am isolierten, schlagenden Herz (Herz-Lungen-Präparat der Katze) untersucht. Wie die Dosis-Wirkungskurven zeigen, ist der direkt negativ inotrope Effekt bei niedrigen und mittleren Konzentrationen (< 1.5 mg/100 ml BV) nicht ausgeprägt, die direkt negativ chronotrope Wirkung zeigt sich sogar erst bei sehr hohen Konzentrationen.
Vergleicht man äquinarkotische Konzentrationen von Etomidate und Hexobarbital, so fällt die erheblich größere therapeutische Breite von Etomidate auf. Trotz weitgehender Konstanz der übrigen Meßgrößen fand sich jedoch eine starke, konzentrationsabhängige Verminderung des aortalen Schlagvolumens nach Etomidate-Applikation, die möglicherweise als Folge einer relativen Zunahme des koronaren Schlagvolumenanteils zu interpretieren ist.

Die myokardiale Adaptationsfähigkeit an definierte Druck- oder Volumenbelastungen ist unter Etomidate weitgehend erhalten, wird jedoch durch äquinarkotische Hexobarbitalkonzentrationen erheblich eingeschränkt. Die vergleichende Studie läßt die Schluß-folgerung zu, daß Etomidate als Einleitungshypnotikum bei Patienten mit eingeschränkter kardialer Leistungsbreite gegenüber gebräuchlichen Substanzen Vorteile haben könnte.

References

1. BARNES, G.E., BISHOP, V.S., HORWITZ, L.D., KASPAR, R.L.: The maximum derivation of left ventricular pressure and transverse internal diameter as indices of inotropic state of the left ventricle in conscious dogs. J. Physiol. (Lond.) 235, 571 (1973).

2. BÖTTCHER, H., FISCHER, K.-J., PROPPE, D.: Untersuchungen über die Wirkung von Digoxigenin- mono-, bis- und -tridigotoxosid am Herz-Lungen-Präparat der Katze. Basic Res. Cardiol. 69, (1974).

3. BRAUNWALD, E., ROSS, J., Jr., SONNENBLICK, E.H.: Mechanism of contraction of the normal and failing heart. Boston: Little & Brown 1968.

4. BRAUNWALD, E.: Myocardial function - 1972. Anesth. Analg. Curr. Res. 51, 489 (1972).

5. BRÜCKNER, J.B., GETHMANN, J.W., PATSCHKE, D., TARNOW, J., WEYMAR, A.: Untersuchungen zur Wirkung von Etomidate auf den Kreislauf des Menschen. Anaesthesist 23, 322 (1974).

6. BRUGMANS, J., JAGENEAU, A., DENEF, B.: Cardiovascular effects of etomidate in normal man. Janssen Res. Prod. Inform. Service (N 8124) (1974).

7. DOENICKE, A., GABANYI, D., LEMCKE, H., SCHÜRK-BÜLICH, M.: Kreislaufver-halten und Myokardfunktion nach drei kurzwirkenden i.v. Hypnotika Etomi-date, Propanidid, Methohexital. Anaesthesist 23, 108 (1974).

8. FISCHER, K.: Die Wirkung von Ketamine auf den Herzmuskel. Anesth. Inform. 12, 187 (1971).

9. FISCHER, K.: Experimentelle Untersuchungen über den Einfluß von Dehydro-benzperidol, Fentanyl bzw. Thalamonal auf die myokardiale Kontraktilität. In: Neuroleptanalgesie. Spezielle Probleme: Einsatz in der nicht-opera-tiven Medizin (Hrsg. W.F. HENSCHEL), S. 27. Stuttgart: Schattauer 1972.

10. FISCHER, K.: Vergleichende tierexperimentelle Untersuchungen zum Einfluß verschiedener Narkotika auf das Herz. Anaesthesiologie und Wiederbelebung, Bd. 69. Berlin-Heidelberg-New York: Springer 1973.

11. FISCHER, K.-J., MARQUORT, H.: Tierexperimentelle Untersuchungen zur Wir-kung von Etomidate auf die Kontraktilität des isolierten, intakten Warm-blüterherzens (Herz-Lungen-Präparat der Katze). Stuttgart: Schattauer 1974.

12. GUYTON, A.C.: Regulation of cardiac output. Anesthesiology 29, 314 (1968).

13. GUYTON, A.C.: Textbook of medical physiology, 4th Ed. Philadelphia: Saunders 1971.

14. HEMPELMANN, G., HEMPELMANN, W., PIEPENBROCK, S., OSTER, W., KARLICZEK, G.:
    Die Beeinflussung der Blutgase und Hämodynamik durch Etomidate bei myocardial vorgeschädigten Patienten. Anaesthesist 23, 423 (1974).

15. HERPFER, G.E.: Über die Messung der Kontraktionsfähigkeit des Herzmuskels.
    Meßmethodische Grundlagen und Problematik. Anaesthesist 19, 35 (1970).

16. HILL, A.V.: The heat of shortening and the dynamic constant of muscle.
    Proc. roy. Soc. B. (Lond.) B. 126, 136 (1938).

17. HUGENHOLTZ, P.G., ELLISON, R.C., URSCHEL, C.W., MIRSKY, I., SONNENBLICK,
    E.H.: Myocardial force-velocity relationships in clinical heart disease.
    Circulation 41, 191 (1970).

18. JAGENEAU, A., XHONNEUX, R., RENEMAN, R.S.: Cardiovascular effects of the
    intravenously injected shortacting hypnotics etomidate, methohexital and
    propanidid in unanesthetized dogs. Janssen Res. Prod. Inform. Service
    (R-26490/3 (1973).

19. JANSSEN, P.A.J., NIEMEGEERS, E.J.E., SCHELLEKENS, K.H.C., LENAERTS, F.M.:
    Etomidate, R-(+)-Ethyl-1-(∝-methyl-benzyl) imidazole-5-carboxylate
    (R 16659) a potent, short-acting relatively atoxic intravenous hypnotic
    agent in rats. Drug. Res. 21, 1234 (1971).

20. KETTLER, D., SONNTAG, H., WOLFRAM-DONATH, U., REGENSBURGER, D., HOEFT,
    H.-J., SCHENK, H.D.: Hämodynamik, Myokardfunktion, Koronardurchblutung
    und Sauerstoffversorgung des Herzens unter Etomidate. Vergleich mit
    anderen intravenösen Narkotika. Stuttgart: Schattauer 1974 a.

21. KETTLER, D., SONNTAG, H., DONATH, U., REGENSBURGER, D., SCHENK, H.D.:
    Hämodynamik, Myokardmechanik, Sauerstoffbedarf und Sauerstoffversorgung
    des menschlichen Herzens unter Narkoseeinleitung mit Etomidate.
    Anaesthesist 23, 116 (1974 b).

22. KÖHLER, E.: Der Einfluß des enddiastolischen Druckes auf die Verkürzungs-
    geschwindigkeit der kontraktilen Elemente des Herzmuskels. Paper presented
    at the 39th meeting of the Dtsch. Ges. Kreislaufforsch., Bad Nauheim
    (1973).

23. KÖHLER, E., MESCHER, H.: Ermittlung ventrikulärer Druck-Geschwindigkeits-
    kurven unter Berücksichtigung des enddiastolischen Druckes. Pflügers
    Arch. ges. Physiol. 342, 83 (1973).

24. KRAYENBÜHL, H.P.: Die Dynamik und Kontraktilität des linken Ventrikels.
    Basel: Karger 1969.

25. KRAYER, O.: Versuche am insuffizienten Herzen. Arch. exp. Path. Pharma-
    kol. 162, 1 (1931).

26. MASON, D.T.: The autonomic nervous system and regulation of cardiovascular
    performance. Anesthesiology 29, 670 (1968).

27. MASON, D.T., SPANN, J.F., jr., ZELIS, R.: Myocardial contractile state
    in hypertrophy and congestive failure in conscious man: determination by
    the maximum velocity of contractile element shortening. Circulation 40,
    Suppl. 3, 141 (1969).

28. MASON, D.T., ZELIS, R., AMSTERDAM, E.A.: Beurteilung der Kontraktilität des menschlichen Herzens. Triangel (Sandoz) 9, 273 (1971).

29. MASON, D.T., ZELIS, R., AMSTERDAM, E.A.: Unified concept of the mechanism of action of digitalis: influence of ventricular function and cardiac disease on haemodynamic response to fundamental contractile effect. In: Basic and clinical pharmacology of digitalis (Ed. B.H. MARKS), p. 206. Springfield, Ill.: C. Thomas 1972.

30. MITCHELL, J.H., WALLACE, A.G., SKINNER, N.S., jr.: Intrinsic effects of heart rate on left ventricular performance. Amer. J. Physiol. 205, 41 (1963).

31. MORGENSTERN, C., ARNOLD, G., HÖLJES, U., LOCHNER, W.: Die Druckanstiegs-geschwindigkeit im linken Ventrikel als Maß für die Kontraktilität unter verschiedenen hämodynamischen Bedingungen. Pflügers Arch. ges. Physiol. 315, 177 (1970).

32. MORGENSTERN, C., GOEBEL, H., LOCHNER, W.: Die Beurteilung der Kontraktili-tät des Herzens. Dtsch. med. Wschr. 97, 1563 (1972).

33. NOBLE, M.I.M., BOWEN, T.E., HEFNER, L.L.: Force-velocity relationship of cat cardiac muscle studied by isotonic and quick release technique. Circulat. Res. 24, 821 (1969).

34. NOBLE, I.M.I.: Problems concerning the application of concepts of muscle mechanics to the determination of the contractile state of the heart. Circulat. 45, 252 (1972).

35. PATTERSON, S.W., STARLING, E.H.: On the mechanical factors which deter-mine the output of the ventricles. J. Physiol. (Lond.) 48, 357 (1914).

36. RAFF, U., STAUBER, W., KISSLING, G.: Die Aussagekraft verschiedener Kontraktilitätsindizes beim Herzen in situ. Basic Res. Cardiol. 69, 58 (1974).

37. SARNOFF, S.J., MITCHELL, J.H.: Control of function of heart. In: Hdb. Physiol., Sect. 2, Circulation, Vol. 1 (Ed. W.F. HAMILTON, P. DOW), p. 489. Washington: Amer. Physiol. Soc. 1962.

38. SCHMIDT, H.D., HOPPE, H., SCHNEIDER, W.: Usefulness of some pressure velocity parameters for evaluation of left ventricular contractility. Paper presented at the 39th meeting of the Dtsch. Ges. Kreislaufforsch., Bad Nauheim 1973.

39. SHIMOSATO, S.: Isovolemic intraventricular pressure change: an index of myocardial contractility during anesthesia. Anesthesiology 31, 327 (1969).

40. SIEGEL, H., SONNENBLICK, E.H.: Quantification and prediction of myocardial failure. Arch. Surg. 89, 1012 (1964).

41. SONNENBLICK, E.H.: Applications of muscle mechanics in the heart. Fed. Proc. 21, 975 (1962 a).

42. SONNENBLICK, E.H.: Force-velocity relations in mammarian heart muscle. Amer. J. Physiol. 202, 931 (1962 b).

43. STRAUBER, B.E.: Kriterien zur Beurteilung der Myokardcontraktilität am
     normalen Herzmuskel. Klin. Wschr. 51, 259, 306 (1973).

44. TARNOW, J., PASSIAN, J., PATSCHKE, D., WEYMAR, A., BRÜCKNER, J.B.:
     Nierendurchblutung unter Etomidate. Anaesthesist 23, 421 (1974).

45. WEYMAR, A., EIGENHEER, F., GETHMANN, J.W., REINECKE, A., PATSCHKE, D.,
     TARNOW, J., BRÜCKNER, J.B.: Tierexperimentelle Untersuchungen zur Wir-
     kung von Etomidate (R 26490-Sulfat) auf den Kreislauf und die myokardiale
     Sauerstoffversorgung. Anaesthesist 23, 150 (1974).

The Influence of R 26 490 (Etomidate Sulfate) on Ventilation and Gas Exchange

B. Marquardt, H. Waibel and J.B. Brückner

Introduction

JANSSEN et al., (1971) first described the new intravenous hypnotic
agent etomidate, belonging to the hypnotics with imidazole-
carboxylate structure. Investigations in animals and humans
(BRÜCKNER et al., 1974; DOENICKE et al., 1973) followed. In comparison with Althesin, ketamine, methohexitone and propanidid,
etomidate caused only minimal side effects on cardiovascular
system (BRÜCKNER et al., 1974). The present study was undertaken
in order to determine the influence of etomidate on ventilation
and gas exchange in geriatric patients.

Materials and Methods

The investigations were carried out in supine position on 30 male
patients undergoing urological surgery (mean age 69 years, range
60 - 84 years, mean body weight 66 kg, range 60 - 100 kg). The
study included patients with normal values (BALDWIN et al., 1948)
of vital capacity, forced exspiratory volume of 1.0 sec and
residual volume measured with a Mijnhardt water sealed spirometer
Volumograph III, and normal oxygen and carbon dioxid blood gas
tensions (RENCK, 1969; SORBINI et al., 1968) measured with calibrated Gas Check AVL electrodes. The ventilatory response to
carbon dioxid was found to be normal in all patients (BATES et
al., 1971; TENNEY, MILLER, 1956). A premedication of pethidine
1.0 mg/kg b.w. promethazine 0.75 mg/kg b.w. and atropine 6 micro-
gram/kg b.w. was given intramusculary one hour before induction
of anaesthesia.

On arrival in the anaesthetic room an indwelling needle was
inserted into a vein on the dorsum of the hand. Arterial pressure
was measured through a teflon cannula in a radial artery connected
directly to a Statham P 23 Db and a Hellige MR 83. The standard
Einthoven electrocardiogram was recorded from conventional limb.
Rectal temperature was measured (10 patients) using a digital
thermistor thermometer. Samples of arterial blood were withdrawn
during each period of measurement (control 1,3,5,7 and 10 min)
and analysed for PO_2, PCO_2, pH and hemoglobin concentration.

A nasal clamp (10 patients) was placed on the nose and the patient
was allowed to breath air to a low-resistance non-rebreathing
valve (M. Planck-Werkstätten). The exspiratory part of the valve
was connected to a calibrated electric Wright spirometer (NUNN
et al., 1962) designed to measure exspired volume breath by
breath. Using a small Douglas bag the mixed exspired gas concentration of oxygen and carbon dioxid were analysed during each

period of measurement (SYKES, MILLER, 1970) with a Hartmann & Braun Oxytest-S and Uras-IV. The total ventilation (V_E) was calculated in ml/min BTPS, the oxygen uptake and carbon dioxid elimination in ml/min STPD. The physiological dead space ventilation (V_{Df}) was determined from the Bohr equation (COMROE et al., (1968). In order to measure the alveolar ventilation ($\dot{V}_A$) it was necessary to subtract the dead space ventilation from the total ventilation.

The calculated dose of etomidate (0.3 mg/kg b.w.) was injected during a period of 45 - 60 sec. and all continuously measured variables were recorded on an 8-channel-recorder (Hellige EK 21). Surgical procedure was not carried out during the investigations. Mean values were calculated for each group and the results analysed by applying the Student-t-test for correlated means to the control values and those for each subsequent minute.

Results

The effect of etomidate on oxygen uptake and carbon dioxid elimination is shown in Fig. 1.

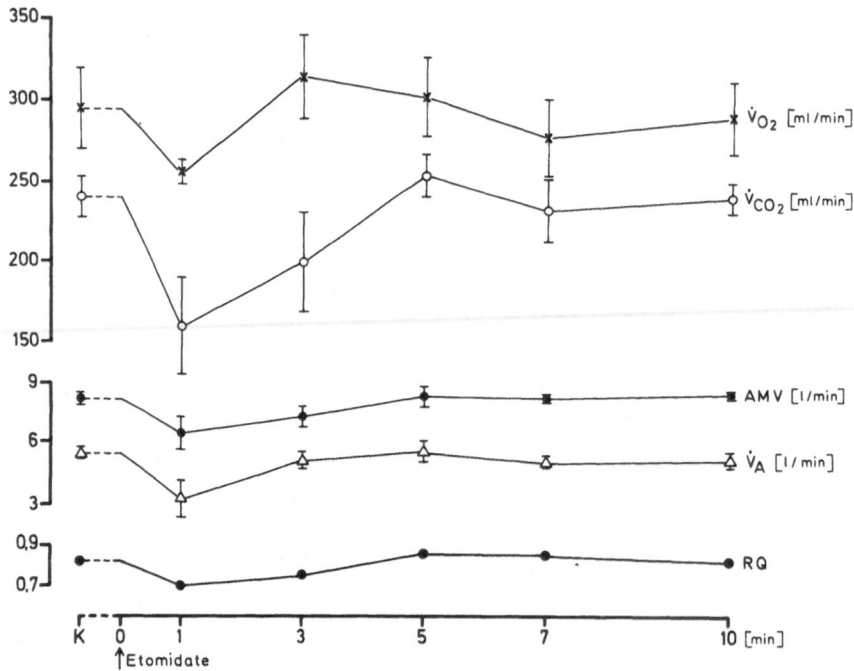

Fig. 1.Changes in oxygen uptake, carbon dioxid elimination, exspired minute volume, alveolar ventilation and respiratory quotient (mean and SD) after injection of 0.3 mg/kg b.w. of etomidate (n = 10)

The minute volume ($\dot{V}_E$) decreased after the 1st minute. The ventilation became irregular caused by decreased tidal volumes ($\dot{V}_E$ control: 7.8 ± 0.34 l/min. $\dot{V}_{E,\ 1}$ 6.454 ± 0.899 l/min BTPS; p< 0.01; 21 % of control; $\dot{V}_{E,\ 3}$ x̄ 7.242 ± 0.525 l/min BTPS; p< 0.05). The respiratory frequency was slightly increased (f control x̄ 15.5 ± 0.48/min; f_1 x̄ 17.4 ± 0.750/min; p< 0.05). During the 5th minute, the control values were reached again. The alveolar ventilation decreased during the 1st minute to the extent of 39 % of control ($\dot{V}_A$ control x̄ 5.8 ± 0.386 l/min; $\dot{V}_{A,\ 1}$ x̄ 3.21 ± 0.89 l/min BTPS; p< 0.05) and was nearly normal during the 3rd minute. The physiological dead space ventilation ($\dot{V}_{Df}$ control x̄ 2.76 ± 0.12 l/min BTPS; 34.6 % of exspired volume) increased significantly during the 1st minute ($\dot{V}_{Df,\ 1}$ x̄ 3.244 ± 0.68 l/min BTPS; p< 0.01) to 50 % of exspired volume during the 5th minute to 43 % and during the 7th minute to 38 % of the total ventilation. Three patients developed an initial apnoe lasting 20 to 25 sec. Oxygen uptake and carbon dioxid elimination decreased with hypoventilation.

The effect of etomidate on arterial blood gases is shown in fig. 2.

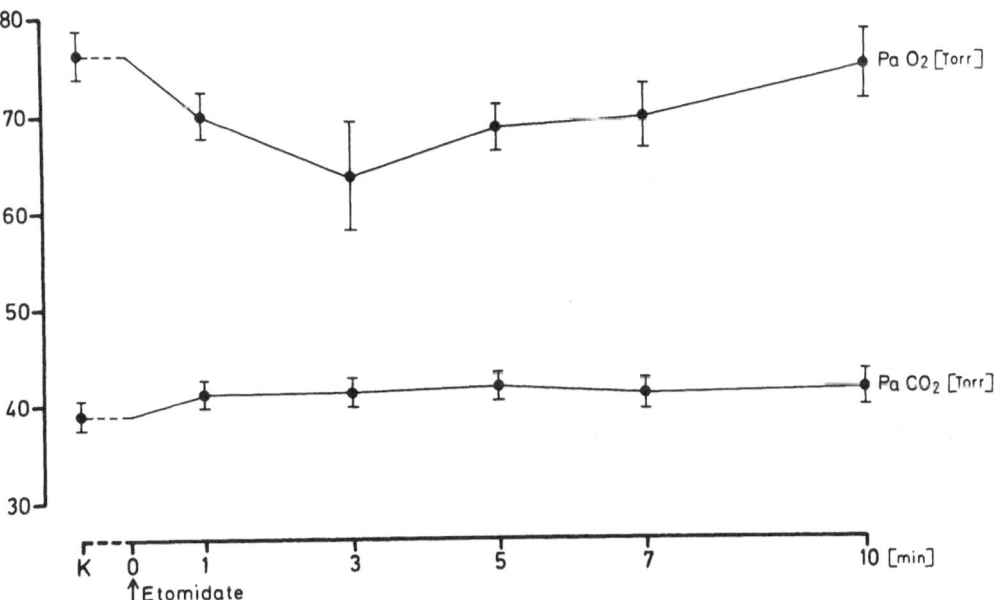

Fig. 2. *Changes of arterial oxygen tension and carbon dioxid tension (mean and SD) after injection of 0.3 mg/kg b.w. of etomidate (n = 20)*

The arterial oxygen tension (PO_2 control $\bar{x}$ 76.2 $\pm$ 8.1 mmHg) decreased during the 1st minute to the extent of 9 % of control ($PO_{2,\ 1}$ $\bar{x}$ 70.2 $\pm$ 2.1 mmHg; $p < 0.01$) and reached the lowest level at the 3rd minute ($PO_{2,\ 3}$ $\bar{x}$ 63.5 $\pm$ 3.6 mmHg; $p < 0.001$). The carbon dioxid tension increased slightly, but not significantly. The mean pH remained unchanged and no marked changes in blood pressure and pulse rate were found. All variables were restored to control values during the 10th minute.
Consciousness returned after 4 min / 41 sec $\pm$ 136 sec.

Discussion

DOENICKE et al., (1973) using doses of 0.15 mg/kg b.w. in young people, reported no significant changes of oxygen and carbon dioxid tension and pH in the arterial blood. In this study a brief period of hypoventilation was seen after 0.3 mg/kg b.w. of etomidate in geriatric patients. The mean minute volume, tidal volume, alveolar ventilation, oxygen uptake, and carbon dioxid elimination decreased while respiratory frequency and dead space ventilation increased. An etomidate induced initial apnoe lasted only 20 to 25 sec. PO_2 decreased significantly, while PCO_2 increase did not reach a significant level. It seems difficult to compare the pharmacological effects of etomidate with other intravenous hypnotic agents because the relative potencies of these drugs have not yet been determined. Propanidid (REICHEL et al., 1965; ZINDLER, 1969) has a biphasic action on respiration. The initial hyperventilation is followed by a period of hypoventilation and sometimes apnoe. An elevation of arterial PCO_2 and dangerous decrease of arterial PO_2 may occur. The respiratory effects of the barbiturates are a result of direct depressant actions on the medullary and pontine representations of respiratory control. At surgical levels of anaesthesia tidal volume is diminished and respiratory rate increased (FEUERSTEIN, 1964; WYANT, CHANG, 1959). The application of barbiturates, propanidid and etomidate was followed by a decrease of PO_2 and an increase of PCO_2.

The respiratory pattern of etomidate looks like the pattern of the barbiturates, but there is no evidence about the same mechanism of action. Etomidate may lead to direct depression of the respiratory center or may alter the ventilation/perfusion ratio caused by myoclonus of the thoracical muscles.
Assisted or controlled ventilation appears to be necessary in geriatric patients after treatment with etomidate (dosage 0.3 mg/kg b.w.)

Acknowledgements

We would like to thank Dr. P.A.J. Janssen of Janssen Pharmaceutica n.v., Beerse/Belgium, for the supply of etomidate (R 26 490), and Mrs. A. Mahlitz and Mrs. R. Rubbert for technical assistance.

Summary

Etomidate is a short acting intravenous anaesthetic agent. After injection of 0.3 mg/kg b.w. in geriatric patients with normal respiratory function it produces a short period of hypoventilation, sometimes apnoe. Arterial oxygen tension decreases noteworthy, while arterial carbon dioxid tension remains unchanged. Poor risk patients should be given oxygen mask with assisted or if necessary controlled ventilation.

Zusammenfassung

Etomidate ist ein kurzwirkendes, intravenöses Anaesthetikum. Nach Injektion von 0,3 mg/kg Körpergewicht bewirkt es bei geriatrischen Patienten eine kurzfristige Hypoventilation, manchmal einen Atemstillstand. Der arterielle Sauerstoffpartialdruck sinkt signifikant, während der arterielle Kohlendioxidpartialdruck unverändert bleibt. Eine assistierte oder kontrollierte Beatmung mit Sauerstoff wird empfohlen.

References

1. BALDWIN, E.F., COURNAND, A., RICHARDS, P.W.: Pulmonary insufficiency I. Physiological classification, clinical methods of analysis standard values in normal subjects. Medicine (Baltimore) 27, 243 (1948).

2. BATES, D.V., MACHLAN, P.T., CHRISTIE, R.V.: Respiratory Function in Disease. Philadelphia-London-Toronto: Saunders 1971.

3. BRÜCKNER, J.B., GETHMANN, J.W., PATSCHKE, D., TARNOW, J., WEYMAR, A.: Studies on the circulatory effects of etomidate in man. Anaesthesist 8, 322 (1974).

4. COMROE, J.H., FORSTER, R.E., DUBOIS, A.B., BRISCOE, W.A., CARSTEN, E.: The Lung. Stuttgart: Schattauer 1968.

5. DOENICKE, A., WAGNER, E., BEETZ, K.H.: Arterial blood gas analyses following administration of three short-acting intravenous hypnotics. Anaesthesist 22, 353 (1973).

6. FEUERSTEIN, V.: In: Intravenous Anaesthesia. International Anaesth. Clinics 2, 740 (1964).

7. JANSSEN, P.A.J., NIEMEGEERS, C.J.E., SCHELLEKENS, K.H.L., LENAERTS, F.M.: Etomidate, a potent short-acting and relatively atoxic intravenous hypnotic agent in rats. Drug. Res. 21, 1234 (1971).

8. NUNN, J.F., EZI ASHI, T.I.: The accuracy of the respirometer and ventigrator. Brit.J.Anaesth. 34, 422 (1962).

9. REICHEL, G., PODLESCH, I., ULMER, W.T., ZINDLER, M.: Untersuchungen über die Wirkung des Kurznarkotikums Propanidid auf Ventilation und Gasstoffwechsel. Anaesthesist 14, 184 (1965).

10. RENCK, H.: The elderly patient after anaesthesia and surgery. Acta anaesth.scand. Suppl. XXXIV (1969).

11. SORBINI, C.A., GRASSI, V., SOLINAS, E., MIESAU, G.: Arterial oxygen tension in relation to age in healthy subjects. Respiration 25, 3 (1968).

12. SYKES, M.K., MILLER, R.M.: Principles of Measurement for Anaesthetics. Oxford-Edinburgh: Blackwell 1970.

13. TENNEY, S.M., MILLER, R.M.: Respiratory response in the age. J. appl. Physiol. 9, 321 (1956).

14. WYANT, G.M., CHANG, C.A.: Sodium methohexital, a clinical study. Cand. Anaesth. Soc. J. 6, 40 (1959).

15. ZINDLER, M.: Changes of respiratory and blood gases after propanidid. Acta anaesth.scand. 17, 67 (1965).

A Comparative Study of Blood Gases and Haemodynamics Using the New Hypnotic Etomidate, CT 1341, Methohexitone, Propanidid, and Thiopentone

W. Hempelmann, G. Hempelmann and S. Piepenbrock

Introduction

The new hypnotic etomidate has been of much interest since its introduction by JANSSEN et al., (1971) and first clinical reports by DOENICKE et al., (1973 a-d; 1974, in press). Haemodynamic investigations in animals (TARNOW et al., 1974; WEYMAR et al., 1974) and man (BRÜCKNER et al., 1974; HEMPELMANN et al., 1974; KETTLER et al., 1974) confirmed that etomidate has only minor effects on most of these parameters. It was our interest to investigate its effect on blood gas parameters in a comparative study using different short acting anaesthetics.

Material and Methods

Induction of anaesthesia has been performed in a total of 76 patients with arteriosclerotic or cardiac diseases using five different induction agents:
etomidate, a new hypnotic; CT 1341 (Althesin), a steroid anaesthetic; methohexitone (Brevimytal), a short acting barbiturate; propanidid (Epontol) and thiopentone (Trapanal), another barbiturate.

Blood pressure, heart rate, and arterial blood gas parameters (pO_2, pCO_2) as well as pH and base excess (BE) have been controlled before and during an 8-minute investigation period. Furthermore, arterial pO_2-monitoring was performed continuously, using a Clark-type flow-through oxygen-electrode (FABEL, 1968; HEMPELMANN et al., 1974) (Fig. 1). During this investigation period the patients were breathing spontaneously ambient air. No infusions or transfusions were given. Injection time in all patients was between 10 and 20 seconds.

Results

1. Etomidate

Etomidate was given to 18 patients using 0.3 mg:kg (first group) or 0.15 mg/kg (second group).

0.3 mg/kg etomidate caused a significant decrease in systolic and diastolic blood pressure (- 15 %) (Fig. 2). In this group of patients with cardiac diseases heart rate decreased from a mean

120

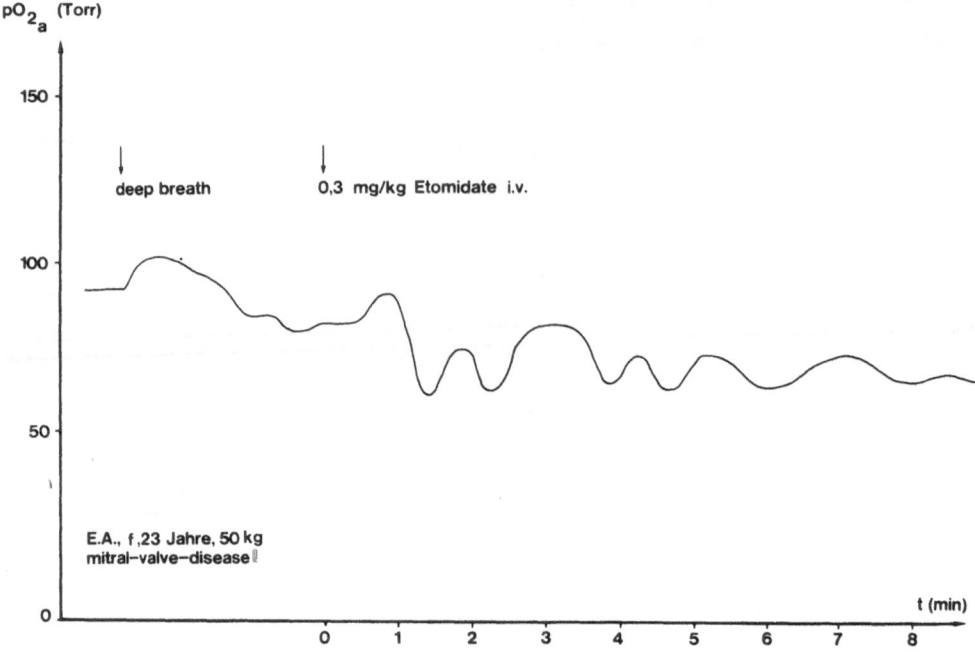

Fig. 1.*Continuously monitored arterial pO$_2$ during induction of anaesthesia using 0.3 mg/kg etomidate*

of 99.9 $\pm$ 11.1 beats per min. to 89.0 $\pm$ 9.7 beats per min.

Arterial pO$_2$ decreased significantly to a minimum of 66.3 $\pm$ 4.0 torr. Three of these patients had arterial pO$_2$-values between 50 and 60 torr for a short period without any haemodynamic complications.

In this group of patients there was, however, no significant difference between the initial pH-, pCO$_2$- and base excess values (7.39 $\pm$ 0.01; 33.4 $\pm$ 1.3 torr; - 3.0 $\pm$ 0.7 meq/l) and the eight-minute control values (7.39 $\pm$ 0.01; 34.0 $\pm$ 1.3 torr; - 3.1 $\pm$ 0.8 meq/l).

0.15 mg/kg etomidate was given to 10 patients with arterio-sclerotic diseases.

Changes in blood pressure and heart rate in this group were only small (Fig. 3): There was an initial decrease in systolic blood pressure by 5 % and later on a small increase by approx. 5 %. Heart rate remained almost constant during the whole investigation period. There were, however, significant changes in arterial pO$_2$: Although pO$_2$ went down below the 60-torr-limit in four patients[2] (Fig. 4), the mean value of the individual pO$_2$-minima was only

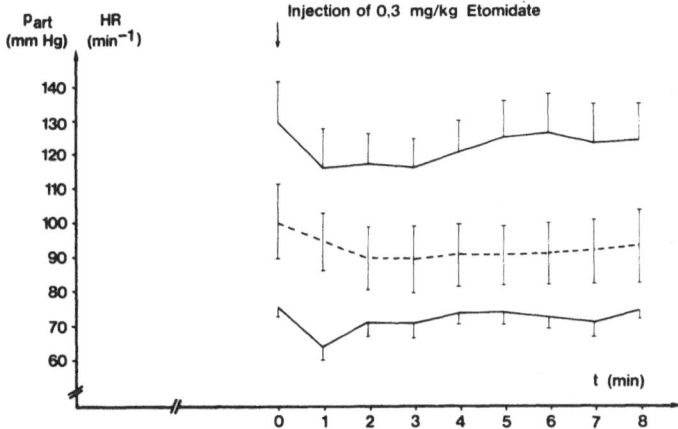

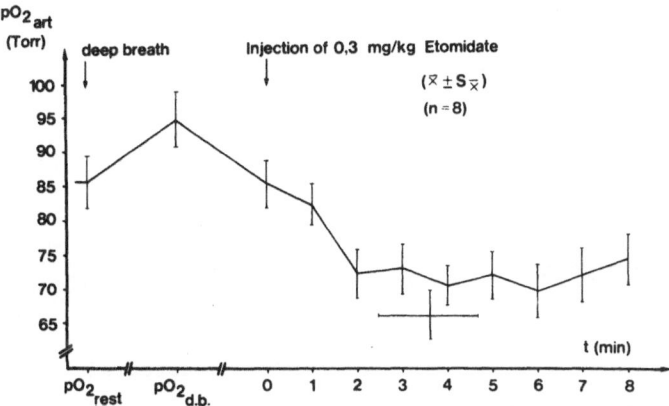

Fig. 2.Mean values of blood pressure (p_{art}), heart rate (HR) and arterial pO_2 ($pO_2\ _{art}$) before and during induction of anaesthesia using 0.3 mg/kg etomidate ($pO_2\ _{d.b.}$ = pO_2 maximum after a deep breath)

61.1 $\pm$ 4.4 torr. Eight minutes after injection of etomidate pO_2 was back to control values. Neither in group 1 (using 0.3 mg/kg etomidate) nor in group 2 (using 0.15 mg/kg etomidate) we could find any significant changes in pCO_2, pH, or base excess when comparing initial values and eight-minute control values. According to the mean age there was a difference in initial pO_2-values: group one (0.3 mg/kg) had a mean age of 41 years and group two (0.15 mg/kg) - only patients with arteriosclerotic diseases - had a mean age of 61 years.

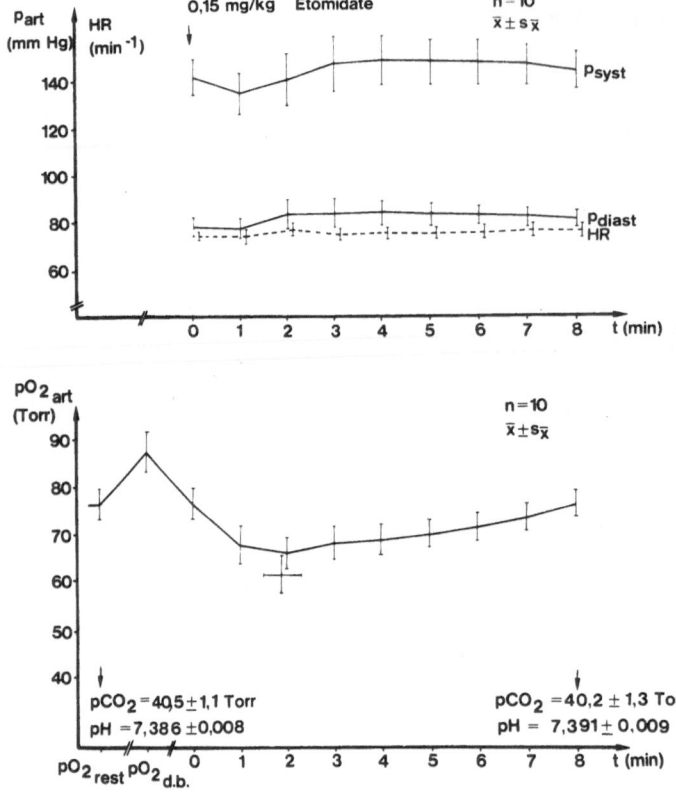

Fig. 3.*Mean values of blood pressure (p_art), heart rate (HR) and arterial*
pO₂ (pO₂ art) in 10 patients before and during induction of anaesthesia using
0.15 mg/kg etomidate

2. CT 1341 (Althesin)

The intravenous steroid anaesthetic Althesin (CT 1341) was given
to 18 patients with arteriosclerotic diseases. Immediately after
the injection of 0.05 ml/kg there was a significant decrease in
blood pressure (- 20 %); heart rate increased by 9 % (Fig. 5).
Continuous arterial pO_2-monitoring demonstrated a decrease from
a mean of 71.4 ± 2.5 torr to a minimum of 46.1 ± 3.0 torr
(P < 0.001). One patient had to be ventilated because of a dramatic
decrease in arterial pO_2 with clinical signs of hypoxia.

3. Methohexitone (Brevimytal)

1 mg/kg methohexitone caused a 10 % decrease in blood pressure
and a 16 % increase in heart rate (Fig. 6). 2 1/2 minutes after
intravenous injection of methohexitone there was a pO_2-minimum
of 52.2 ± 2.2 torr (p < 0.001). Seven minutes after injection mean
arterial pO_2-values were above the 60-torr-limit.

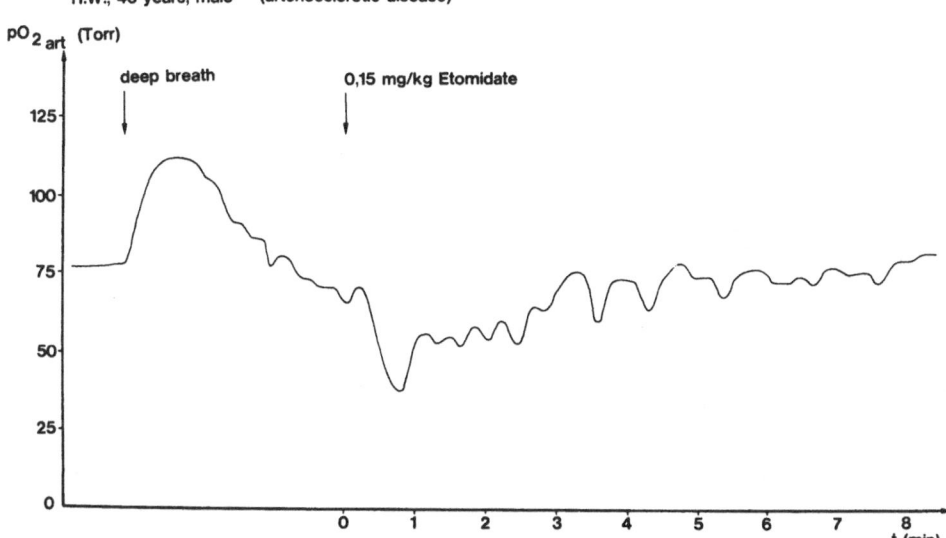

Fig. 4.Continuously monitored arterial pO₂ during induction of anaesthesia in a patient with arteriosclerotic disease using 0.15 mg/kg etomidate

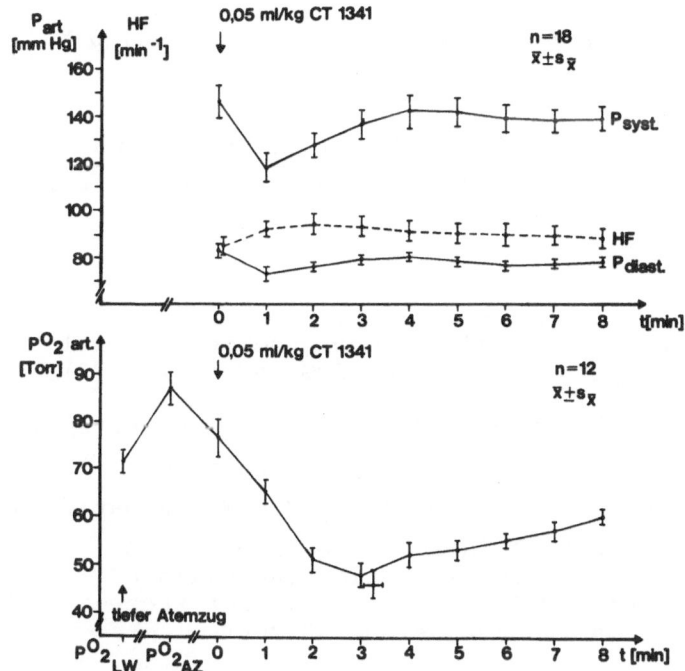

Fig. 5.Mean changes in blood pressure (p_{art}), heart rate (HR) and arterial pO₂ during induction of anaesthesia using 0.05 ml/kg CT 1341 (Althesin)

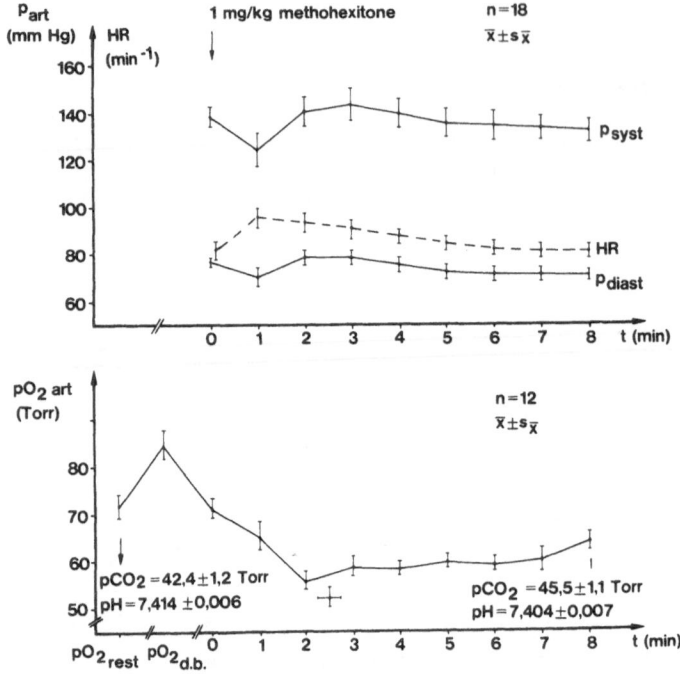

Fig. 6.Changes in blood gas parameters and haemodynamics after injection of 1 mg/kg methohexitone (Brevimytal)

There was a slight increase in arterial pCO_2-values at the end of the investigation period (45.5 $\pm$ 0.9 torr) compared to control values (42.6 $\pm$ 1.0 torr).

4. Propanidid (Epontol)

Anaesthesia with propanidid leads to a 30 % decrease in arterial blood pressure and an increase in heart rate (SOGA et al., 1972).

The arterial pO_2-curves were characterized by a typical hyperventilation effect with a rise in pO_2 initially and a subsequent decrease in pO_2 because of hypoventilation (Fig. 7). In 12 patients 4 mg/kg propanidid caused an initial increase in arterial pO_2 (91.9 $\pm$ 3.8 torr); 3 1/2 minutes after induction there was a minimum of 60.8 $\pm$ 2.7 torr (p<0.001) (Fig. 8). Five of these patients had minimal pO_2-values between 54 and 48 torr.

5. Thiopentone (Trapanal)

In 10 patients 4 mg/kg thiopentone caused an initial drop in blood pressure (- 14 %) and an increase in heart rate (+ 9 %) (Fig. 9).

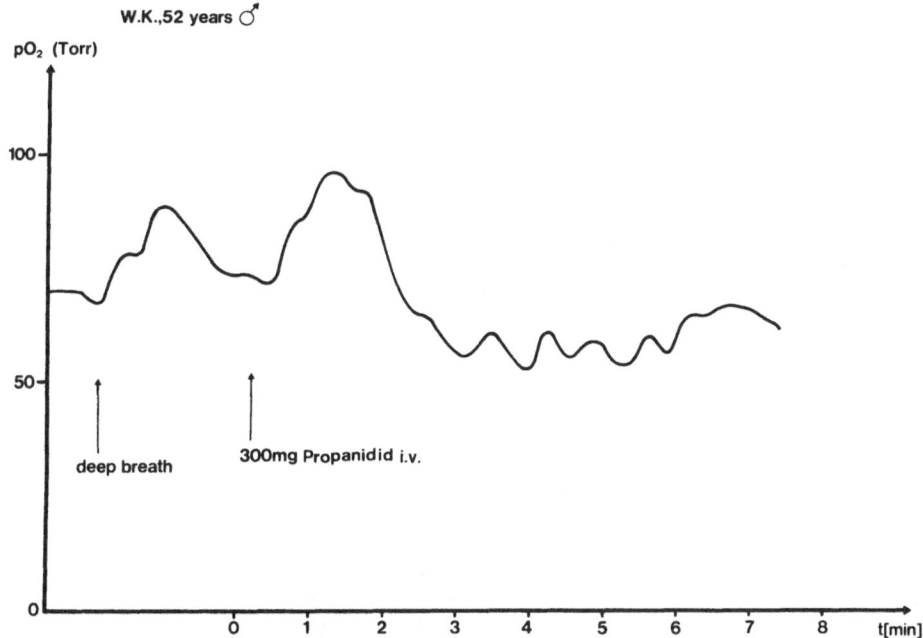

Fig. 7. Continuously monitored arterial pO₂-curve: Induction of anaesthesia in a patient with 4 mg/kg propanidid (Epontol)

Arterial pO_2 went down continuously to a minimum of 45.9 ± 3.0 torr 3 1/2 minutes after induction. One patient had to be ventilated because of a decrease in partial pressure to a minimum of 37.4 torr; clinical signs of hypoxia and ectopical beats disappeared immediately after ventilation with oxygen. Nine of the patients in this group had a pO_2-minimum below 55 torr and 5 of these even below 45 torr. At the end of the investigation period pO_2-values were significantly lower and pCO_2-values higher than control values.

Discussion

Our investigations demonstrate, that there is a severe decrease in arterial pO_2, when using thiopentone and CT 1341. Mean pO_2-values in the methohexitone-group were slightly below the 60-torr-limit (Fig. 10). During induction with propanidid and etomidate mean changes in partial pressure were lesser than in the other three groups. Nevertheless, etomidate as well as propanidid cause a significant decrease in arterial pO_2, which can lead to hypoxic periods in patients, which is confirmed by recent investigations (MARQUARDT et al., in press). In contrast to DOENICKE et al., (1973) we could find no increase in arterial pO_2 when

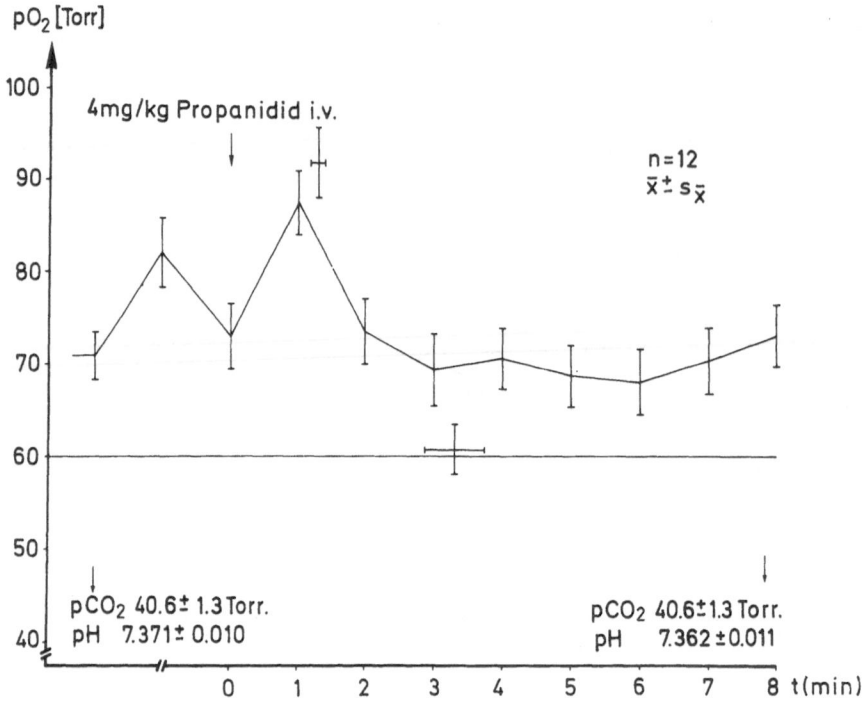

Fig. 8.*Mean changes in arterial blood gas parameters after injection of 4 mg/kg propanidid (Epontol) in a group of 12 patients*

using etomidate, neither in group one (0.3 mg/kg) nor in group two (0.15 mg/kg).

Arterial pCO_2-values increased in the thiopentone-, Althesin- and methohexitone-group. There was, however, no significant difference in pCO_2-values in the propanidid- and etomidate-groups 8 minutes after injection, compared to control values (HEMPEL-MANN et al., 1973).

Our haemodynamic investigations confirm, that propanidid, CT 1341, and thiopentone can cause severe haemodynamic changes, especially in patients with cardiovascular diseases (HEMPELMANN et al., in press). Methohexitone and etomidate seem to have lesser effects on haemodynamics (BRÜCKNER et al., 1974; HEMPELMANN et al., 1974; SOGA et al., 1972).

Although we know that etomidate is only a hypnotic agent without any relevant analgetic effect, we think that it is a safer drug for induction of anaesthesia than propanidid, CT 1341, or thiopentone.

Our continuous arterial pO_2-monitoring demonstrated that there is no induction agent without any negative effects on arterial pO_2-

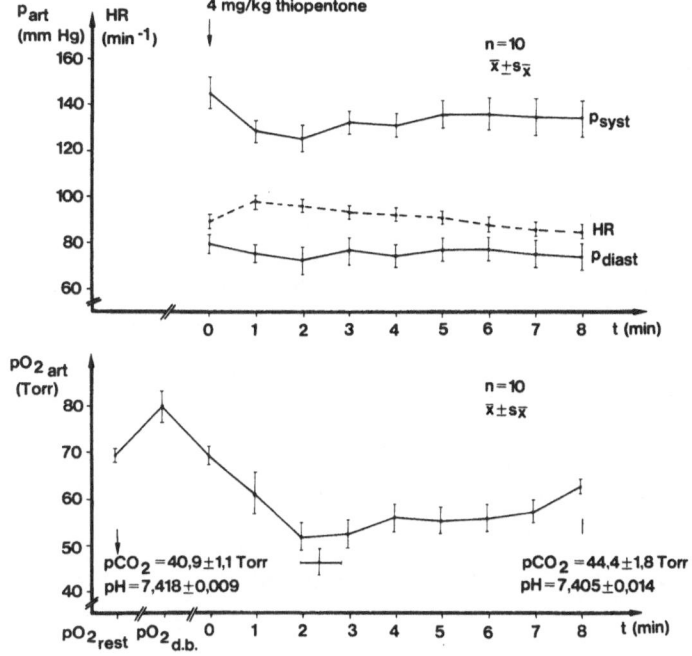

Fig. 9. Mean changes in blood pressure (p_{art}), heart rate (HR) and arterial pO_2 during induction of anaesthesia using 4 mg/kg thiopentone (Trapanal)

values. Therefore any induction of anaesthesia should be performed using oxygen and - if necessary - assisted ventilation must be at hand.

Summary

A comparative study of blood gas parameters and haemodynamics was performed in 76 patients using five different agents: etomidate, Althesin (CT 1341), Brevimytal (methohexitone), Epontol (propanidid) and Trapanal (thiopentone).
According to these investigations etomidate has only minor effects on arterial blood gas parameters and haemodynamics; it seems to be the drug of choice for induction of anaesthesia, especially in high risk patients.

Zusammenfassung

In einer vergleichenden Untersuchung an insgesamt 76 Patienten wurde der Effekt von fünf verschiedenen Narkoseeinleitungsmitteln auf arterielle Blutgase, den Säure-Basen-Haushalt sowie hämo-dynamische Parameter festgestellt.
Aufgrund dieser Ergebnisse läßt sich sagen, daß Etomidate nur geringfügige Veränderungen hervorruft; es scheint - insbesondere bei Risikopatienten - das Mittel der Wahl zur Narkoseeinleitung zu sein.

128

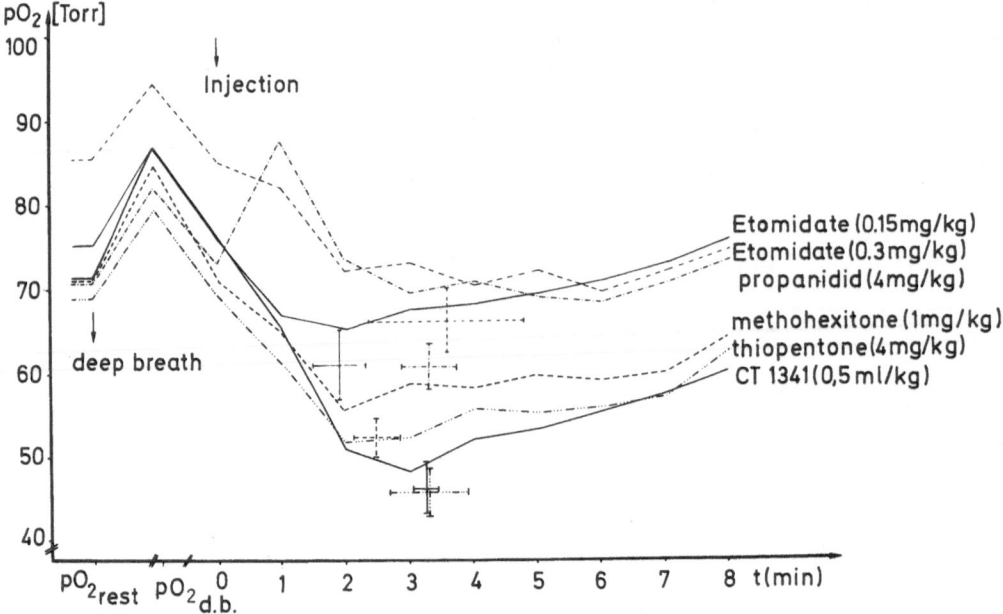

Fig. 10.Mean changes in arterial pO_2 after injection of different induction agents (crosses indicate mean value of the pO_2-minimum from every patient in the different groups, respectively)

References

1. BRÜCKNER, J.B., GETHMANN, J.W., PATSCHKE, D., TARNOW, J., WEYMAR, A.: Untersuchungen zur Wirkung von Etomidate auf den Kreislauf des Menschen. Anaesthesist 23, 322 (1974).

2. DOENICKE, A.: Klinisch-experimentelle Untersuchungen und klinischer Erfahrungsbericht über ein neues i.v. applizierbares Narkotikum. 6. Internationaler Fortbildungskurs für klinische Anaesthesiologie. Wien, 21.-25. Mai 1973. Tagungsbericht (1973).

3. DOENICKE, A., KUGLER, J., PENZEL, G., LAUB, M., KALMAR, J., KILLIAN, I., BEZECNY, H.: Hirnfunktion und Toleranzbreite nach Etomidate, einem neuen barbituratfreien i.v. applizierbaren Hypnotikum. Anaesthesist 22, 357 (1973).

4. DOENICKE, A., KALMAR, L.: Die Aufgaben des Anaesthesisten bei der Erprobung neuer Anaesthetica. Wandertagung; Ungarische Gesellschaft für Anaesthesiologie und Reanimation, Debrecen, August 1973. Tagungsbericht (1973).

5. DOENICKE, A., KUGLER, J., LORENZ, W., WAGNER, E., LEMCKE, H., KALMAR, L., PRAETORIUS, B. SCHELLENBERGER, A., SCHUNDINGER, ST., SPIESS, W.: Experimentelle Untersuchungen und klinische Erfahrungen mit dem neuen i.v. Kurznarkotikum Etomidate. Vortrag XIII. Gemeinsame Tagung der Deutschen, Schweizerischen und Österreichischen Gesellschaften für Anaesthesiologie und Wiederbelebung. Bd. 93, 149. Berlin-Heidelberg-New York: Springer 1975.

6. DOENICKE, A., WAGNER, E., BEETZ, K.H.: Blutgasanalysen (arteriell) nach drei kurzwirksamen i.v. Hypnotika (Propanidid, Etomidate, Methohexital). Anaesthesist 22, 353 (1973).

7. DOENICKE, A., GABANYI, D., LEMCKE, H., SCHÜRK-BULICH, M.: Kreislaufverhalten und Myocardfunktion nach drei kurzwirksamen i.v. Hypnotika: Etomidate, Propanidid, Methohexital. Anaesthesist 23, 108 (1974).

8. FABEL, H.: Die fortlaufende Messung des arteriellen Sauerstoffdruckes beim Menschen. Arch. Kreisl.-Forsch. 57, 145 (1968).

9. HEMPELMANN, G., HARTMANN, W., FABEL, H.: Fortlaufende Messungen des arteriellen Sauerstoffdrucks. Anwendungsmöglichkeiten und Beispiele aus der Anaesthesie. Anaesthesiologie und Wiederbelebung, 80. Berlin-Heidelberg-New York: Springer 1974.

10. HEMPELMANN, G., HEMPELMANN, W., PIEPENBROCK, S.: Vergleichende Untersuchungen über fortlaufende arterielle pO_2-Messungen und Kreislaufkontrollen bei Kurznarkosen mit CT 1341, Methohexital, Propanidid und Thiobarbiturat. Langenbecks Arch. Chir., Supplement, 1973.

11. HEMPELMANN, G., HEMPELMANN, W., PIEPENBROCK, S., OSTER, W., KARLICZEK, G.: Die Beeinflussung der Blutgase und Hämodynamik durch Etomidate bei myokardial vorgeschädigten Patienten. Anaesthesist 23, 423 (1974).

12. HEMPELMANN, G., KARLICZEK, G., PIEPENBROCK, S.: Hämodynamische Untersuchungen bei über 100 herzchirurgischen Patienten unter Verwendung von 10 verschiedenen Narkoseverfahren. Jahrestagungder Deutschen Gesellschaft für Anaesthesie und Wiederbelebung, Erlangen, 1974. Erlangen: Perimed, Kongreßband, S. 951.

13. JANSSEN, P.A.J., NIEMEGEERS, C.J.E., SCHELLEKENS, K.H.L., LENAERTS, F.M.: Etomidate, R(+)Ethyl-1-(alpha-methyl-benzyl)imidazole-5-carboxylate (R 16659), a potent, shortacting relatively atoxic intravenous hypnotic agent in rats. Arzneimittel-Forsch. 21, 1234 (1971).

14. KETTLER, D., SONNTAG, H., DONATH, U., REGENSBURGER, D., SCHENK, H.-D.: Hämodynamik, Myokardmechanik, Sauerstoffbedarf und Sauerstoffversorgung des menschlichen Herzens unter Narkoseeinleitung mit Etomidate. Anaesthesist 23, 116 (1974).

15. MARQUARDT, B., WAIBEL, H., BRÜCKNER, J.B.: Der Einfluß von R 26 490 (Etomidate-Sulfat) auf Ventilation und Gasaustausch. Excerpta Medica, Amsterdam-London: 1975.

16. SOGA, D., BEER, R.: Myocardkontraktilität und Hämodynamik im Verlauf einer Methohexital-Narkose. In: LEHMANN, CH.: Anaesthesiologie und Wiederbelebung, Bd. 57. Berlin-Heidelberg-New York: Springer 1972.

17. TARNOW, J., PASSIAN, J., PATSCHKE, D., WEYMAR, A., BRÜCKNER, J.B.: Nierendurchblutung unter Etomidate. Anaesthesist 23, 421 (1974).

18. WEYMAR, A., EIGENHEER, F., GETHMANN, J.W., REINECKE, A., PATSCHKE, D., TARNOW, J., BRÜCKNER, J.B.: Tierexperimentelle Untersuchungen zur Wirkung von Etomidate (R 26490-Sulfat) auf den Kreislauf und die myokardiale Sauerstoffversorgung. Anaesthesist 23, 150 (1974).

The Use of Etomidate as an Induction Agent in Fentanyl Analgesia

Z. Kalenda

Introduction

The trend in the development of anaesthetic techniques over the
years has been towards minimal narcosis, maximal muscular relaxation and maximal stability of the autonomic nervous system.

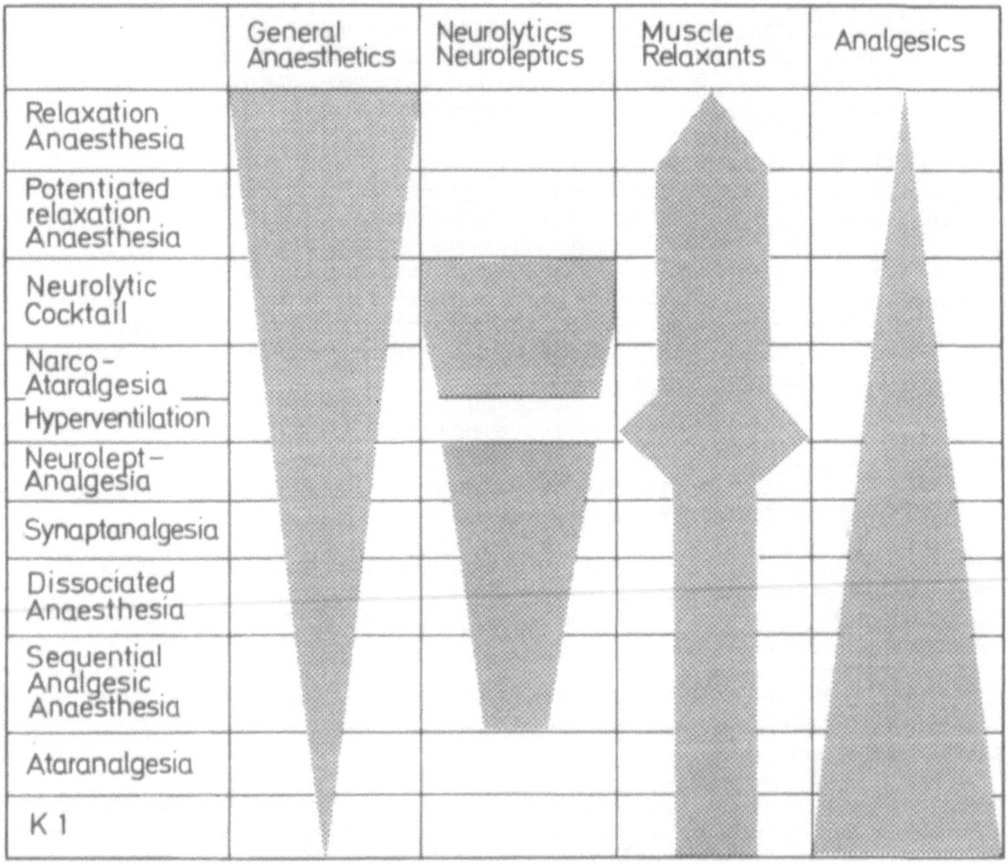

	General Anaesthetics	Neurolytics Neuroleptics	Muscle Relaxants	Analgesics
Relaxation Anaesthesia				
Potentiated relaxation Anaesthesia				
Neurolytic Cocktail				
Narco-Ataralgesia Hyperventilation				
Neurolept-Analgesia				
Synaptanalgesia				
Dissociated Anaesthesia				
Sequential Analgesic Anaesthesia				
Ataranalgesia				
K 1				

Fig. 1.The changing role of the pharmacological components

DE CASTRO and MUNDELEER made the first significant step towards
autonomic stabilization when they introduced NLA in 1959. The
powerful centrally acting analgesic, fentanyl, was found to be
the pharmacological keystone in this technique. In 1968 DE CASTRO
and VIARS eliminated neuroleptics and used large doses of fentanyl

alone, reversing the end-respiratory depression with pentazocine. He called this technique "sequential analgesic anaesthesia" (DE CASTRO, VIARS, 1968). In 1970 he abandoned the use of an antidote and placed the patient on a respirator until the respiratory depressant effects had worn off. This he called "ataranalgesia" (DE CASTRO, 1972).

Fig. 1 is an illustration of the changing emphasis on each of the four major components which have been used in anaesthesia. Powerful general anaesthetic drugs have declined to vanishing point, as have neurolytics and neuroleptics in some circles. Muscle relaxants still play an important role, but analgesia is becoming the focal point because in proportion to its potency it provides autonomic stability and thus eliminates the effects of damaging reflexes.

Some years ago, we became interested in the obvious and latent potentialities of these ideas and we began to work along similar lines. Our first modification was the use of etomidate as an induction agent. We preferred its rapid onset, its broad safety margin and brief duration of action as compared with those of the longer-acting hypnotics dinitrofluorazepam and rohypnol, which, in our hands, frequently resulted in prolonged post-operative narcosis.

Methods

Our present technique has been standardized as follows (dosages refer to the average patient): The patient receives a sedative (5 mg nitrazepam) the night before operation. Premedication consists of 1 1/2 ml Thalamonal i.m. and 0.5 mg atropine i.m., 30 - 40 min before induction.

Anaesthesia is induced by the rapid injection of 0.5 mg (10 ml) fentanyl, immediately followed by the fairly rapid intravenous injection of 15 mg etomidate. Muscle relaxation for intubation is obtained with 40 mg suxamethonium. After intubation the patient is ventilated with nitrous oxide and oxygen (3 : 1 l/min), using a Servo-ventilator 900. As soon as the suxamethonium is seen to have worn off a non-depolarizing muscle relaxant is injected. We prefer dextrotubocurarine chloride but in about 30 % of cases we used pancuronium bromide.

The duration of the effect of 0.5 mg fentanyl is strikingly constant, namely 50 - 55 min on average, for both analgesia and autonomic stability. Therefore, the moment to give the next increment is predictable. This is fortunate since the drug wears off with startling suddenness. Each increment of 0.5 mg fentanyl i.v. is combined with approx. 10 mg tubocurarine i.v. Repeated injections of fentanyl have been given up to a total dose of 8 mg over a period of 15 hours without detectable side effects.

As the patients are given assisted ventilation at the end of the operation, we consider it unnecessary to reverse the relaxants. Generally the patients wake up and respond to commands as soon as

the nitrous oxide is discontinued. The tube is left in situ and
the patient is ventilated manually during transport to the recov-
ery-room where he is connected to a respirator with a good trigger
mechanism. Provided that hypercapnia is prevented and triggering
is efficient, the patient invariably settles down immediately.
Actually most of the patients (73 %) begin to breathe spontaneously
as soon as they wake up but, in the absence of any stimulus, they
fall asleep again and stop breathing.

Fig. 2 shows a capnogram taken at the end of an operation when
the patient is on the respirator (AR). When the respirator is
switched off, the patient wakes up and at once begins to breathe
(SR), but soon he falls asleep again and stops breathing. Such
a phenomenon is called pseudo-periodic respiration.

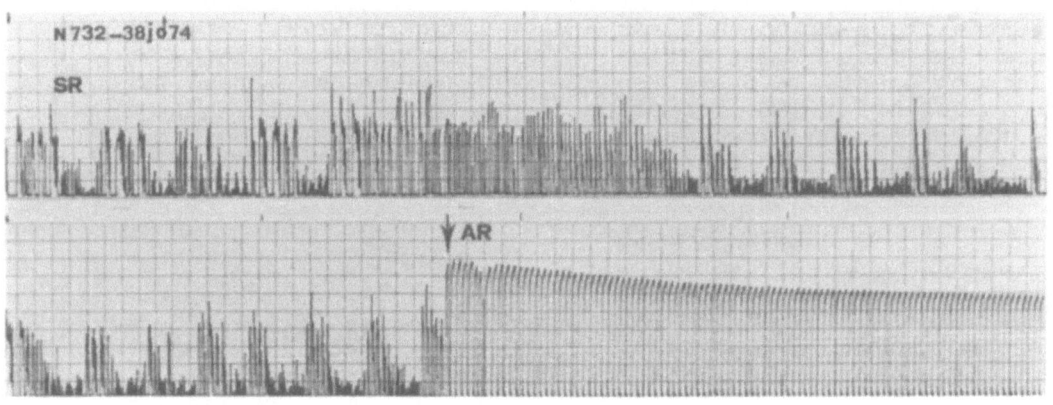

*Fig. 2.Pseudo-periodic respiration caused by the patient falling asleep. The
percentage CO_2 in the expired air as determined by capnography is shown.
AR = artificial respiration; SP = spontaneous respiration. 1 large vertical
division = 1 %; 5 large horizontal divisions = 1 min*

A capnogram taken during true periodic respiration shows a per-
fectly regular cycle, which is controlled by the changing level
of the CO_2 (Fig. 3). This type of respiration was never seen
following our technique.

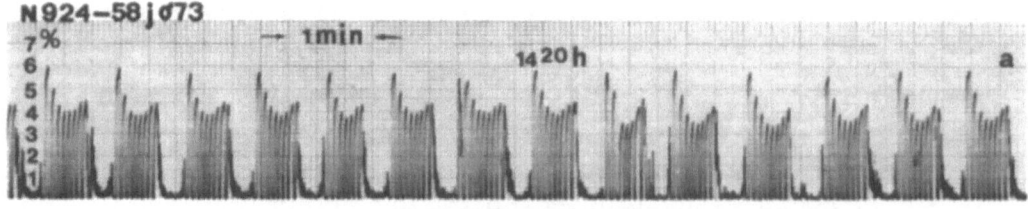

*Fig. 3 True periodic respiration (CHEYNE, STOKES). The percentage CO_2 in the
expired air as determined by capnography is shown. 1 large vertical division
= 1 %; 5 horizontal divisions = 1 min*

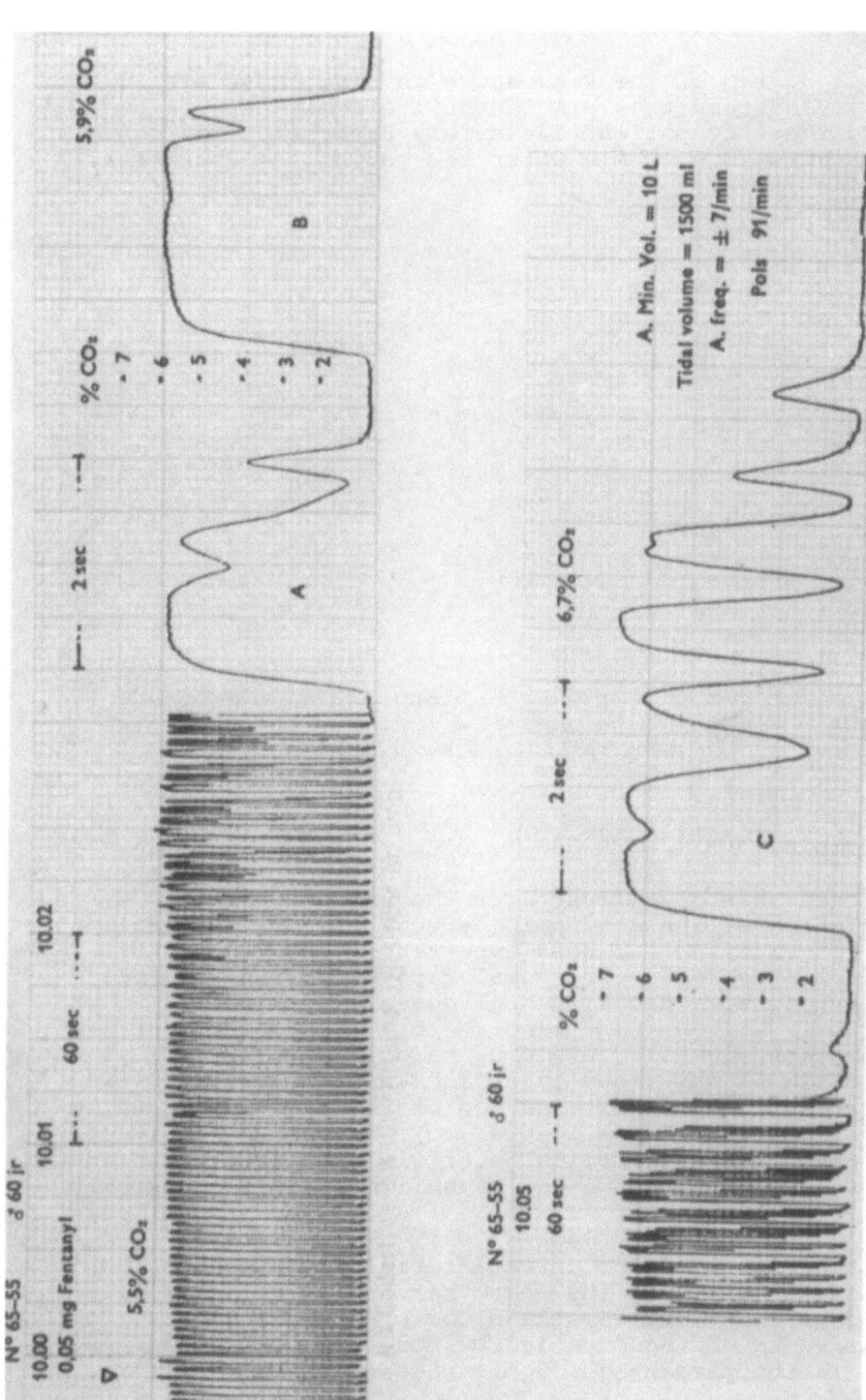

Fig. 4.Effect of fentanyl on capnogram during spontaneous respiration; fast and slow recording speeds. The percentage CO_2 in the expired air is shown (after SMALHOUT B., 1967). 1 large vertical division = 1 %. 5 large horizontal divisions = 1 min (slow speed) or 2 sec (fast speed)

A classical capnogram of spontaneous respiration influenced by
fentanyl is shown in Fig. 4. The fast recording speed has been
used to show 4 individual breaths.

As soon as a capnogram of the kind shown in Fig. 5 has been
obtained, we are certain that all fentanyl-effects have been
eliminated and that the patient can safely breathe on his own.
Usually this occurs 30 - 60 min after the end of the operation.

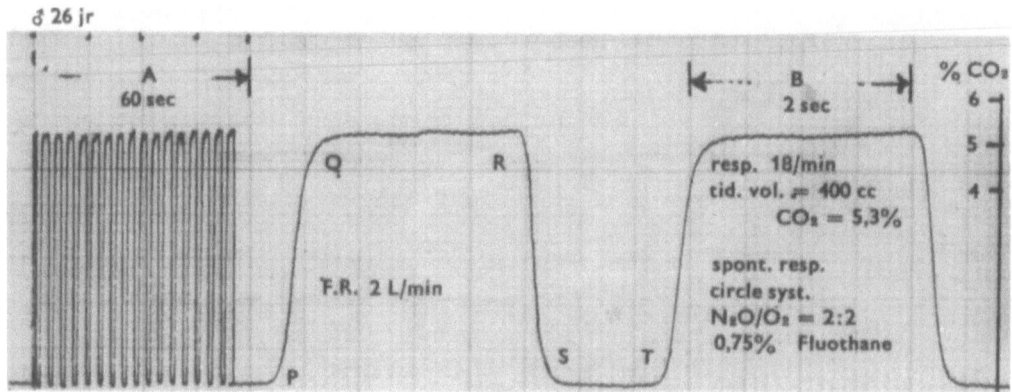

Fig. 5. Normal capnogram during spontaneous respiration. The percentage CO_2
in the expired air is shown. 1 large vertical division = 1 %; 5 large
horizontal divisions = 1 min (slow speed) or 2 sec (fast speed)

A Clinical Example

The following case history illustrates the unique stability during
extreme stimulation of the autonomic nervous system. The patient
was a boy of 16 years who had been hypertensive for a long time.
He suffered from attacks of paroxysmal tachycardia and had been
treated with hypotensive drugs in high doses.

Contrast radiography revealed a glomus caroticum tumour. His signs
and symptoms could be explained by an increase in the level of
circulating catecholamines. Extirpation of the tumour was anatom-
ically impossible. The alternative was to make the tumour inactive
by injecting, into its pathological nutrititional artery, an inert
polymeric substance with the object of obliterating the vascular
bed.

Fig. 6 shows the effect of the intra-arterial injection of the
inert substance. In spite of the fact that the circulating catecholamines had risen 600 times, the blood pressure only rose to
its pre-operative level, accompanied by moderate tachycardia and
a slight rise in the percentage CO_2 in the expired air. After a
few minutes, heart rate, arterial blood pressure and the percentage
CO_2 in the expired air, returned to the original pre-injection

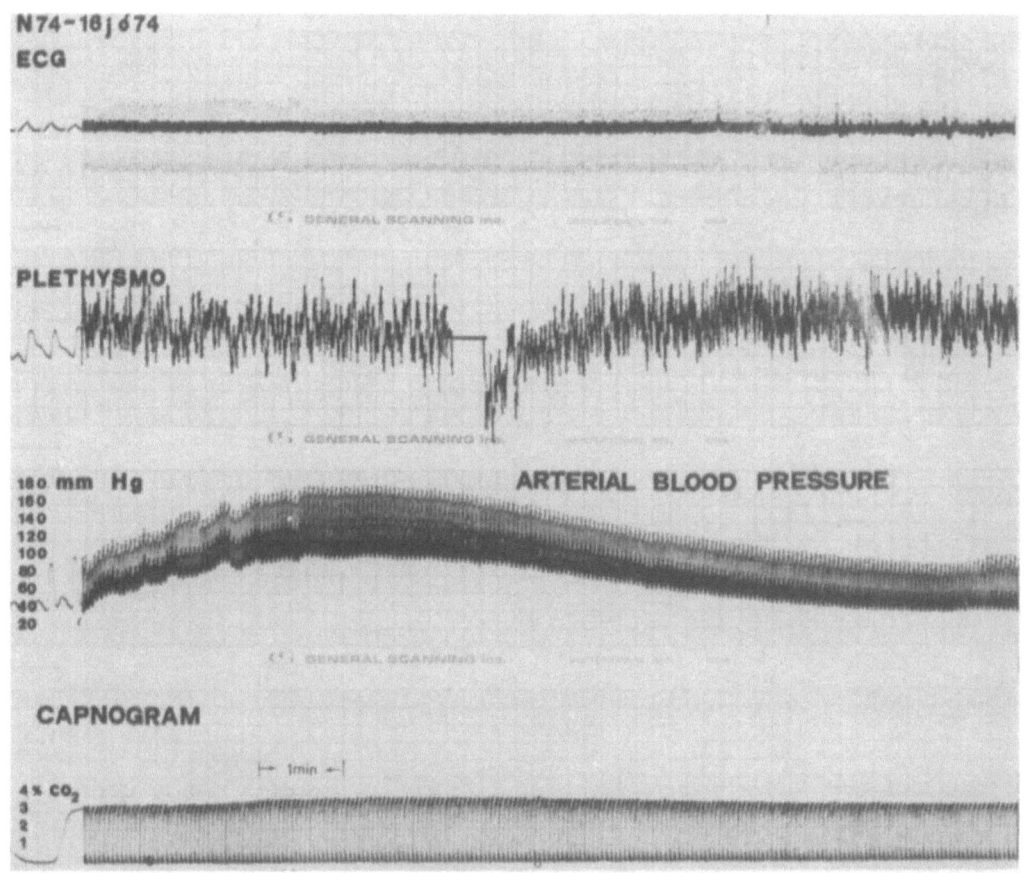

Fig. 6.The effect of the injection of an inert substance into the pathological nutritional-artery on ECG, plethysmogram, arterial blood pressure and capnogram in a patient of 16 years with a glomus caroticum tumour

levels. No severe hypotension occurred afterwards, as is the case with other types of anaesthesia. Hypotension is usually seen after a fall in the circulating catecholamines.

Discussion

We have used this technique in 307 patients during major surgical procedure such as laminectomies. The mean duration of operation was 217 min. (range: 50 - 975 min).

The major advantages of our technique are:

1. The stability of analgesia and anaesthesia in operations of long duration (Fig. 7).
2. Pharmacological simplicity.
The anaesthetist's complete armamentarium is reduced to four drugs. Fentanyl provides deep analgesia and the most complete

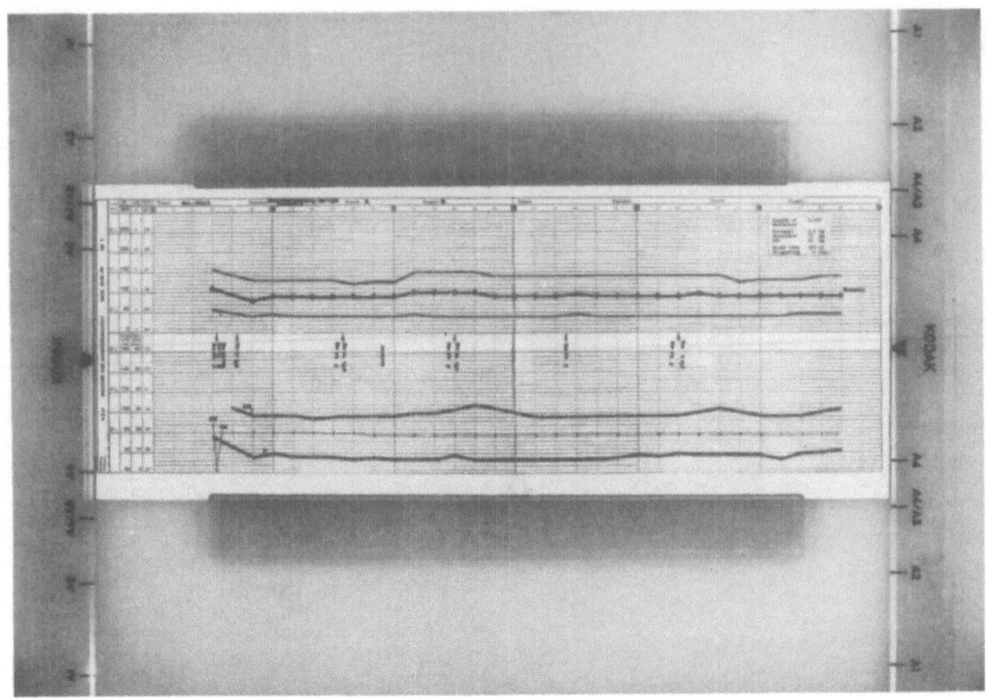

Fig. 7.Oscillometer deflections (first, maximum and last oscillation), percentage CO_2 in the expired air and pulse frequency (P) during an operation
of more than 5 hours. F = fentanyl, E = etomidate, Sux = suxamethonium,
dT_C = d-tubocurarine, SR = spontaneous respiration, CR = controlled respiration.
Postoperative assisted-ventilation was required for 14 min

autonomic stability yet attainable. Anaesthesia is induced
by etomidate and maintained by nitrous oxide. Muscular relaxation is achieved by non-depolarizing muscle relaxants. No
supplementary drugs of any kind e.g. α- and ß-blockers are
required.

3. Simplicity of management
    The effects of the few drugs used are easy to supervise and
    control.
4. Smooth post-operative course.
    Analgesia is maintained until the end of the third day.
5. Perfect operating conditions
    with minimal bleeding; as a result of the autonomic stability.

The disadvantages are:

1. Need for rigorous post-operative monitoring, assisted venti-
    lation and skilled supervision.
2. Low doses of fentanyl can cause vomiting and this level is
    reached as elimination of the analgesic proceeds. Dehydro-
    benzperidol 2 1/2 - 5 mg (1 - 2 ml) will control and prevent

this provided it is given before vomiting has occurred.
Increased salivation is a reliable indication.

This technique is especially indicated for:

1. Operations of longer duration.
2. Anaesthesia in poor risk patients.
3. Operations in which instability of the autonomic nervous
    system is anticipated, e.g. extirpation of phaeochromocytoma
    and endocrinologically active tumours of the glomus caroticum.

Contra-indications are:

1. Patients addicted to morphine and morphinomimetics.
2. Caesarian section.
3. Inadequate equipment and lack of experienced personnel.
4. Pre-existing central respiratory depression or when this
    depression can be expected to occur, e.g. in craniotomies.
5. Children, because of our present lack of knowledge with
    regard to this age group.
6. Operations of short duration.

Summary

The author reviews the development of anaesthesia over the years
and up to the present day, with the current emphasis on increasing
analgesia and the stability of the autonomic nervous system. He
describes a technique which he considers to be a significant
advance in this direction.

After intravenous induction with etomidate he uses large doses
of fentanyl together with muscle relaxants, nitrous oxide and
oxygen. The maximum dose of fentanyl used was 8 mg during a 15
hours operation.

Such a degree of autonomic stability is achieved that during an
operation on a glomus tumour, in which the circulating catecholamines were shown by assay to have increased 600 times, heart
rate and blood pressure were only insignificantly affected.

Most patients awoke as soon as the nitrous oxide was discontinued
and breathed spontaneously, but if left undisturbed, they "forgot
to breathe" and apnoea occured. Respiratory control was guided
by capnography and the patients were put on a respirator with an
efficient trigger mechanism until all signs of fentanyl effect
had disappeared. This guaranteed that the patient could be safely
extubated and sent back to the ward, normally after 30 - 60 min.

Zusammenfassung

Der Autor gibt einen Überblick über die Entwicklung der Anaesthesie
vom Anfang bis zur heutigen Technik, wobei die Analgesie eine
stets mehr bedeutende Rolle spielt und die Stabilität des autonomen
Nervensystems betont wird. Er beschreibt weiter eine Technik,

138

die seiner Meinung nach einen signifikanten Fortschritt in dieser Richtung bedeutet.

Nach intravenöser Anaesthesieeinleitung mit Etomidate verwendet er hohe Fentanyldosen zusammen mit Muskelrelaxanzien, Lachgas und Sauerstoff. Die höchste Fentanyldose während einer 15 Stunden dauernden Operation war 8 mg. Die erzielte autonome Stabilität ist so hoch, daß bei einem wegen Glomustumor operierten Patienten, dessen zirkulierende Katecholamine um 600 mal zugenommen hatten, Herzfrequenz und Blutdruck nur unbedeutend beeinflußt wurden.

Die meisten Patienten erwachten gleich bei Ausschaltung der Lachgaszufuhr und atmeten spontan. Wenn sie jedoch nicht angeregt wurden, "vergaßen sie zu atmen" und es entstand Apnöe. Die Atmung wurde kapnografisch kontrolliert und die Patienten wurden an einen Atemapparat mit einem zuverlässigen Auslösemechanismus angeschaltet, bis jedes Zeichen der Fentanylwirkung abgeklungen war. Dadurch wurde garantiert, daß der Patient ohne Gefahr extubiert und - im Durchschnitt 30 bis 60 Minuten später - wieder zum Krankensaal gebracht werden konnte.

References

1. CAMPAN, L.: Diazepam et Narco-ataralgésie. Analg. Anaesth. franç. 7, spec. 1, 193 (1966).

2. DE CASTRO, J., MUNDELEER, P.: Anesthésie sans sommeil "La neuroleptanalgésie". Acta chir. belg. 58, 689 (1959).

3. DE CASTRO, J., MUNDELEER, P.: Anesthésie sans barbituriques: la neuroleptanalgésie. Anaest. Analg. Curr. Res. 16, 1022 (1959).

4. DE CASTRO, J.: S.N.A. à base de fortes doses de Thiamine. Médicine et Hygiène 23, 1012 (1965).

5. DE CASTRO, J.: S.N.A. nostro orientamento attuale, A.T.A.R.O. Symposium S.N.A., Udine 1967.

6. DE CASTRO, J., VIARS, P.: L'utilisation pratique des analgésiques majeurs en anesthésie et réanimation. ARS Medici, Nivelles Belgique, numéro spécial, 18e congres national français d'anesthésie-réanimation, Nantes 6-9 juin 1968.

7. DE CASTRO, J.: Atar-analgesia with RO5-4200, pancuronium and fentanyl or ketamine. Proc. 5th World Congress Anaesthesiology, Kyoto. Amsterdam: Excerpta Medica 1972.

8. DU CAILAR, J.: Narcoataralgésie et O_2, A.A.F. 7, spec. 1, 31, 1966.

9. CORSSEN, G., DOMINO, E.F.: Dissociated anaesthesia. Anaest. Analg. Curr. Res. 45, 29 (1966).

10. GEDDES, I.C., GRAY, T.C.: Hyperventilation for the maintenance of anaesthesia. Lancet 1959 II, 4.

11. GRAY, T.C., HALTON, J.A.: "A Milestone in Anaesthesia?" Proc.roy.Soc.Med. <u>39</u>, 400 (1946).

12. HAYWARD BUTT, J.J.: Ataralgesia: operations without anaesthesia. Lancet <u>1957 II</u>, 972.

13. LABORIT, H.: L'Anesthésie facilitée par les synergies médicamenteuses. Paris: Masson 1971.

14. LABORIT, H., HUGENARD, P.: Pratique de l'hibernothérapie en clinique et en médicine. Paris: Masson 1954.

15. NEFF, W.B. et al.: Potentiated relaxation anaesthesia. Calif.Med. 66, 70 (1947).

16. SMALHOUT, B.: Ademdepressie door fentanyl. In: Capnografie (A. Oosthoek, Ed.), Utrecht: Uitgeversmaatschappy N.V. 1967.

17. SMALHOUT, B., KALENDA, Z.: An Atlas of capnography. Kerckenbosch: Zeist 1975.

Etomidate Anaesthesia for Cardioversion

A. Weymar, D. Patschke, J. Tarnow and J.B. Brückner

Provided that vagal stimulation, antifibrillatory pharmacotherapy, and ß-receptor blockade fail, electrical cardioversion is the treatment of choice in cardiac arrhythmias. Therapeutic reliability has grown substantially since the introduction of DC-defibrillation controlled by the cardiac action cycle (KOUWENHOVEN et al., 1954; LOWN et al., 1962, 1964; MC DONALD et al., 1964), as opposed to AC-defibrillation (ALEXANDER et al., 1961; ZOLL et al., 1956).

As electrical shock is accompanied by painful or unpleasant sensation because of muscle contraction, it is desirable to perform cardioversion under light general anaesthesia. Experience has shown, that low-level anaesthesia with amnesia is sufficient for this short procedure (GRIMM and BACHMANN, 1973; ROTH, 1969; STÖCKER AND HAGER, 1969; STOCK, 1963).

Inhalation anaesthetics like Halothane or Penthrane are unsuitable because of their negative inotropic effect in higher concentration. Furthermore, simultaneous application of sympathomimetics can aggravate existing cardiac arrhythmias (JOHNSTON and NISBET, 1961), and in many patients breathing through the mask is an additional psychological stress-factor.

There are, of course, disadvantages in intravenous anaesthetics, as well. In order to induce a hypnotic stage rapidly, the initial dosage has to be relatively high, which in turn produces a marked depressive side-effect on the heart, obviously undesirable in patients with impaired cardiac function.

For a long time the short-acting non-barbiturate propanidid was advocated as the drug of choice. Today we know that the negative inotropic action of propanidid is almost as prominent as that of the thiobarbiturates. Therefore, it is contraindicated in cardiac risk patients (SOGA et al., 1973).

The new non-barbiturate hypnotic etomidate seems to have suitable pharmacological properties, i.e.: its action is short, patients regain consciousness rapidly, and there are no relevant effects on the cardiovascular system (BRÜCKNER et al., 1973, 1974; DOENICKE et al., 1974; JANSSEN et al., 1971; RENEMAN et al., 1974; WEYMAR et al., 1974 a, 1974 b).

Therefore, we performed cardioversion in 30 patients under etomidate anaesthesia with permanent oscilloscopic observation and registration of the ECG. The blood pressure was also monitored continuously. Most of the patients were suffering from atrial fibrillation or fluttering with absolute arrhythmia, either after operative correction of valvular disease or in degenerative myocardial disease.

Patients were fasting, except in emergencies. After 5 minutes of oxygen-inhalation we injected etomidate-sulfate (Janssen GmbH Düsseldorf, West Germany) within 30 seconds into a vein of the fore-arm. The dosage of etomidate varied between 0.2 and 0.3 mg/kg and was determined by the patients' general condition and the state of his circulation. If the first therapeutic attempt was unsuccessful, a further dose (0.1 - 0.2 mg/kg) of etomidate was injected for a second cardioversion. Breathing was spontaneous, oxygen being provided via the mask. Depending on the individual circulatory time, the onset of anaesthesia occured 1 - 2 min after the injection of etomidate. The current-shock could then be triggered by the R-spike of the ECG. Conversion to sinus rhythm was successful in 26 cases after one or two electrical shocks, the intensity being between 100 and 400 w.-sec. In 6 cases there were initial A-V-dissociation, A-V-rhythm, or ventricular extra-systoles that only changed into sinus rhythm after a while. 5 - 7 min after the injection patients had recovered consciousness. All patients confirmed complete amnesia, they appreciated the method of anaesthesia employed.

We could neither observe circulatory depression nor stimulation, even after repeated injections of etomidate. Since etomidate is the only short-acting intravenous hypnotic until now that does not induce histamine release (DOENICKE et al., 1973), circulatory accidents of the type described with propanidid are not to be expected (LORENZ and DOENICKE, 1973). In contrast to the induction of anaesthesia with barbiturates, patients do not show any after-effects like drowsiness with etomidate. Recovery and early ambulation following the procedure within 30 minutes were always observed. The lack of pre-medication in 90 % of patients resulted in slight muscular movements in 28 % of patients. Muscular movements are typical for etomidate, but do not interfere with the procedure of cardioversion.

We conclude, that etomidate has proved as an useful mono-anaesthetic for 30 cardioversions. This drug seems to have advantages over propanidid because of lesser side-effects on circulation.

Summary

1.   In 30 patients, most of them (90 %) without pre-medication, cardioversion was performed with etomidate intravenously.

2.   0,2 - 0,3 mg/kg of etomidate were sufficient to provide a hypnotic state for 3 to 5 min, during which cardioversion could be performed.

3.   No change in blood-pressure and heart rate was observed after etomidate-injection.

4. In 67 % of patients sinus rhythm was established after the first cardioversion. In 33 % of the patients several shocks and repeated doses (0.1 - 0.2 mg/kg of etomidate) were required.

Zusammenfassung

1. Bei 30 unprämedizierten Patienten wurde eine Kardioversion in einem Etomidate-Schlaf durchgeführt.

2. 0,2 - 0,3 mg/kg Etomidate waren ausreichend zur Erzeugung eines 3 - 5minütigen Schlafstadiums, während dessen die Kardioversion erfolgte.

3. Blutdruck- und Herzfrequenzalterationen als Folge der Etomidate-Injektion wurden nicht beobachtet.

4. Bei 67 % der Patienten trat sofort nach der ersten Kardioversion Sinusrhythmus auf. Bei 33 % der Patienten wurde mehrfach defibrilliert, so daß eine Wiederholungsdosis von 0,1 - 0,2 mg/kg Etomidate erforderlich war.

References

1. ALEXANDER, S., KLEIGER, R. LOWN, B.: Use of external electric countershock in the treatment of ventricular tachycardia. J.Amer.med.Ass. 177, 916 (1961).

2. BRÜCKNER, J.B., GETHMANN, J.W., PATSCHKE, D., TARNOW, J., WEYMAR, A.: Untersuchungen zur Wirkung von Etomidate auf den Kreislauf des Menschen. Anaesthesist 23, 322 (1974).

3. BRÜCKNER, J.B., GETHMANN, J.W., PATSCHKE, D., TARNOW, J., WEYMAR, A.: Etomidate - ein neues intravenöses Anaesthetikum - Kreislaufwirkungen am Menschen und erste klinische Erfahrungen. Vortrag, gehalten auf der 13. Gemeinsamen Tagung der Deutschen, Schweizerischen und Österreichischen Gesellschaft für Anaesthesiologie und Reanimation, Linz/Österreich 1973.

4. DOENICKE, A., LORENZ, W., BEIGEL, R., BEZECNY, H., KALMAR, L., PRAETORIUS,B., UHLIG, G.: Histaminfreisetzung nach kurzwirkenden Narkotika (Althesin CT 1341, d-Etomidate, Epontol und Cremophor EL). Anaesthesist 22, 367 (1973).

5. DOENICKE, A., GABANYI, D., LEMCKE, H., SCHURK-BULICH, M.: Kreislaufverhalten und Myokardfunktion nach drei kurzwirkenden i.v. Hypnotika Etomidate, Propanidid, Methohexital. Anaesthesist 23, 108 (1974).

6. GRIMM, H., BACHMANN, K.: Epontol-Narkose zur Kardioversion. Anaesthesiologie und Wiederbelebung 74, 363 (1973).

7. JANSSEN, P.A.J., NIEMEGEERS, C.J.E., SCHELLEKENS, K.H.L., LENAERTS, F.M.: Etomidate, R-(+)-Ethyl-1-(ᾱ-methyl-benzyl) imidazole-5-carboxylate (R 16 659) a potent, short-acting relatively atoxic intravenous hypnotic agent in rats. Arzneimittel-Forsch. (Drug Res.) 21, 1234 (1971).

8. JOHNSTON, M., NISBET, H.I.A.: Ventricular arrhythmia during halothane anaesthesia. Brit.J.Anaesth. 33, 9 (1961).

9. KOUWENHOVEN, W.B., MILNOR, W.R.: Treatment of ventricular fibrillation using a capacitor discharge. J.app.Physiol. 7, 253 (1954).

10. LORENZ, W., DOENICKE, A.: Biochemie und Pharmakologie der Histamin-freisetzung durch intravenöse Narkosemittel und Muskelrelaxantien. Anaesthesiologie und Wiederbelebung, Bd. 74. Berlin-Heidelberg-New York: Springer 1973.

11. LOWN, B., NEUMANN, I., AMARASINGHAM, R., BERKOVITS, B.V.: Comparison of alternating current with direct current electroshock across the closed chest. Amer.J.cardiol. 10, 223 (1962).

12. LOWN, B., KLEIGER, R., WOLF, G.: The technique of cardioversion. Amer. Heart J. 67, 282 (1964).

13. MC DONALD, L., RESNEKOV, L., O,BRIEN, K.: Direct-current shock in treatment of drug resistant cardiac arrhythmias. Brit.med.J. 1, 1468 (1964).

14. ROTH, I.: Narkose bei Kardioversion. Schweiz.med.Wschr. 99, 1551 (1969).

15. RENEMAN, R.S., XHONNEUX, R., JAGENEAU, A.H.M., HEYKANTS, J., LADURON, P: The pharmacology of etomidate, a new potent, short-acting intravenous hypnotic. Janssen Research Laboratories, Beerse/Belgium. Vortrag Etomidate-Kolloquium, Düsseldorf 1974.

16. SOGA, D., BEER, R., BADER, B., ANDRAE, J., GÖTZ, E.: Die Beeinflussung der linksventrikulären Muskelkontraktilität und Hämodynamik durch Propanidid beim Menschen. Anaesthesiologie und Wiederbelebung Bd. 74. Berlin-Heidelberg-New York: Springer 1973.

17. STÖCKER, L., HAGER, W.: Die Anaesthesiemethoden bei der elektrischen Kardioversion. Anaesthesist 18, 5 (1969).

18. STOCK, J.R.: Cardioversion without anaesthesia (letter to the Editor) New England J.Med. 269, 534 (1963).

19. WEYMAR, A., EIGENHEER, F., GETHMANN, J.W., REINICKE, A., PATSCHKE, D., TARNOW, J., BRÜCKNER, J.B.: Tierexperimentelle Untersuchungen zur Wirkung von Etomidate (R 26 490-Sulfat) auf den Kreislauf und die myocardiale Sauerstoffversorgung. Anaesthesist 23, 150 (1974).

20. WEYMAR, A., HESS, W., PASSIAN, J., PATSCHKE, D., TARNOW, J., BRÜCKNER, J.B.: Hämodynamische Veränderungen bei intravenöser Dauerinfusion von Etomidate. Vortrag auf dem Internationalen Symposium über Probleme der intravenösen Anaesthesie in Bremen 1974.

21. ZOLL, P.M., PAUL, M.H., LINENTHAL, A.J., NORMAN, L.R., GIBSON, W.: The effects of external electrical currents on the heart. Control of cardiac rhythm and induction and termination of cardiac arrhythmias. Circulation 14, 745 (1956).

Etomidate and Fentanyl for Emergency Anaesthesia in Acute Bleeding with Haemorrhagic Shock

M. Zindler

We have been using etomidate in several hundred patients, mainly for short procedures in combination with Fentanyl (incisions of abscesses, removal of drains and packs, cardioversion etc.), and during the induction of neuroleptanaesthesia.

In my experience the most convincing advantage was the use of etomidate in emergency anaesthesia in acute bleeding with haemorrhagic shock. In combination with intermittent doses of fentanyl and nitrous oxide, I recommend etomidate as the method of choice.

I want to illustrate this with a case report:
A 66 years old male patient with the history of mild hypertension, cardiac arrhythmia and coronary insufficiency came first to the Department of Cardiology with the admission diagnosis of myocardial infarction, and was then transferred to surgery with suspected ruptured aneurysm of the abdominal aorta. Since 2 hours before admission no blood pressure could be measured.
After administration of human albumin and blood 1.5 l and 150 ml sodium bicarbonate 6 %, radial artery pressure recovered to 90, pulse rate to 60. Anaesthesia was started with pancuronium 6 mg, 0.3 mg Fentanyl, and sleep was induced by 0.18 mg/kg etomidate. The begin of controlled ventilation resulted in a drop of arterial pressure to 60. It recovered to 100 after 4 doses of each 25 mcg orciprenalin (Alupent) and after endotracheal intubation with lidocain spray the pressure rose to 150. Then N_2O 50 % and intermittend small doses of fentanyl were added. Venous pressure raised to normal, and blood replacement was judged to be adequate, but the cautious dose of 2.5 mg droperidol caused again a drop of the arterial pressure to 60. From the abdominal cavity, 3.5 l of blood were aspirated. It was difficult to find the source of the arterial bleeding, a small tumor adjacent to the liver.

During the 3 hour procedure 6 l of blood and 2 l of fresh plasma were given, and a total dose of 0.65 mg of fentanyl. After a stormy postoperative course with disseminated intravascular coagulation, "shock lung syndrome" requiring mechanical ventilation for 7 days, short lasting renal failure, temporary psychosis, the patient recovered well and was discharged on the 15th postoperative day to the Cardiology Department for further observation and treatment of his cardiac arrhythmia.

Retrospectively it was estimated that at induction of anaesthesia the blood volume deficit was about 1.5 - 2 l. It is believed that an induction of anaesthesia with a barbiturate would have caused a very dangerous or even fatal drop in blood pressure.

Summary

This case report with successful emergency anaesthesia in abdominal haemorrhage and the experimental evidence in dogs (WEYMAR et al., 1974) and in man (KETTLER et al., 1974) that etomidate has no depressive effect on the heart and the circulation leads to the suggestion that induction of anaesthesia with pancuronium, Fentanyl and etomidate followed by nitrous-oxide and supplementary doses of Fentanyl is the method of choice for emergency anaesthesia in acute bleeding with haemorrhagic shock.

Zusammenfassung

Bei einem Patienten mit Verdacht auf ein rupturiertes abdominales Aortenaneurysma wurde mit Pancuronium 6 mg, Fentanyl 0,3 mg und Etomidate 0,18 mg/kg die Narkose eingeleitet und mit Lachgas 50 % und Fentanyl fortgesetzt.

Nach Eröffnung der Bauchhöhle wurden 3,5 l Blut abgesaugt, das von einer arteriellen Blutung eines Adenoms der Leber stammte. Es wurde retrospektiv geschätzt, daß bei der Narkoseeinleitung ein Defizit von etwa 1,5 - 2 l Blut bestand.

Da experimentelle Untersuchungen beim Hund (WEYMAR et al., 1974) und beim Menschen (KETTLER et al., 1974) zeigten, daß Etomidate keine depressive Wirkung auf die Herz- und Kreislauffunktion hat und aufgrund des erfolgreichen Verlaufs dieses Falles, werden die hier verwendeten Mittel als Methode der Wahl empfohlen, wenn für eine Notfalloperation wegen akuter Blutung im hämorrhagischen Schock eine Narkose sofort eingeleitet werden muß.

References

1. KETTLER, D., SONNTAG, H., DONATH, U. REGENSBURGER, D., SCHENK, H.D.: Hämodynamik, Myokardmechanik, Sauerstoffbedarf und Sauerstoffversorgung des menschlichen Herzens unter Narkoseinleitung mit Etomidate. Anaesthesist $\underline{23}$, 116 (1974).

2. WEYMAR, A., EIGENHEER, F., GETHMANN, J.W., REINECKE, A., PATSCHKE, D., TARNOW, J., BRÜCKNER, J.B.: Tierexperimentelle Untersuchungen zur Wirkung von Etomidate (R 26 490-Sulfat) auf den Kreislauf und die myokardiale Sauerstoffversorgung. Anaesthesist $\underline{23}$, 150 (1974).

Clinical Experience with Etomidate in Diagnostical Interventions and Operations of Short Duration

A. Doenicke, W. Spiess, B. Grote and J. Aranoji

In spring 1972, when etomidate was used in clinical practice for the first time, we anaesthetized 5 of 25 patients with the new substance for interventions of short duration. Myocloni as well as an increase in heart-rate, defensive movements during the intervention and other signs of insufficient anaesthesia induced us not to use etomidate anymore as a mononarcotic in subsequent clinical trials (DOENICKE, KUGLER, 1972).

As a result of these observations we tested etomidate in various combinations, which appeared to be pharmacologically useful, in a number of clinical and experimental trials for their anaesthetical suitability in operations of short duration (Table 1).

Table 1. Variation of Premedication

Premedication					Narcotic
Atropin 0.5 mg					
Atropin 0.5 mg + Fentanyl	0.05	-	0.15	mg	Etomidate 15 mg
Atropin 0.5 mg + Thalamonal	1	-	2	ml	Etomidate 15 mg
Atropin 0.5 mg + Diazepam	3	-	7.5	mg	Etomidate 15 mg
Atropin 0.5 mg Diazepam	3	-	7.5	mg	
+				)	Etomidate 15 mg
Fentanyl	0.05	-	0.15	mg	

None of the patients of this study received i.m. premedication. Only comparable interventions of short duration have been evaluated. We always injected atropine i.v. several minutes prior to other drugs. Additional substances were given 1 - 2 min before etomidate.

With fentanyl alone we obtained sufficient analgesia, myocloni were reduced in number and severity, but not fully eliminated.

The combination with Thalamonal was favourable in respect of analgesia and the reduction of myocloni, but unsuitable for out-patients because of possible neuroleptic after-effects lasting from 6 - 8 hours, as we observed in volunteers in a different trial.

Diazepam only reduced the incidence and severity of myocloni (DOENICKE et al., 1973) but had no analgetic effect, so that this combination was not suitable for surgical interventions.

The combination with diazepam and fentanyl appeared to be much more favourable. Patients went quietly to sleep, there were only occasional defensive movements and absolutely no signs of vegetative pain; postoperative recovery was pleasant.

To objectify our clinical experience we conducted comparative studies in volunteers (Table 2).

Table 2. 8 Volunteers

Etomidate	0.30 mg/kg b.w. for induction, subsequent injection after 5 to 12 minutes (0.30 mg/kg b.w. each)
Premedication	a) Atropin 0.5 mg
	b) Atropin 0.5 mg + 1 ml Thalamonal
	c) Atropin 0.5 mg + 0.1 mg/kg b.w. Diazepam

Circulatory system, myocardial function, E.E.G.

Among the Thalamonal/etomidate group two volunteers showed a transient respiratory depression, however, without assisted ventilation becoming necessary. When being questioned 2 hours after anaesthesia 6 of 8 volunteers did not feel fit to drive. Six of these volunteers stated they would not undergo this type of anaesthesia again, because they suffered from an agonizing restlessness lasting from 6 to 8 hours.

On the other hand, volunteers found anaesthesia with etomidate alone or with a combination of etomidate/diazepam quite pleasant and were willing to repeat it any time. They furthermore considered themselves to be fit to drive.

The number of myocloni was about the same in group b and c (Table 2).

The EEG record showed that sleep with diazepam in combination with etomidate was deeper and lasted longer for one to two minutes (DOENICKE et al., 1973).

Apart from EEG control and the circulatory and myocardial function test we considered the traffic fitness test to be very important for out-patient anaesthesia (DOENICKE, KUGLER, 1975).

A combination method (Table 3) to test the efficiency and ability to concentrate, which has successfully been used in our department for the past 12 years already, was now applied in 10 volunteers in study IX; the a.m. method comprises the track-tracer, the labyrinth test according to CHAPIUS, the figures test, the determination device (KIEL), and the KLT counting test by DÜKER.

In this double-blind study (Table 4) each of 10 volunteers underwent one anaesthesia with etomidate 0.3 mg/kg b.w. combined with

0.15 mg fentanyl and diazepam 0.1 mg/kg b.w. as premedication and a <u>second</u> one with etomidate alone, i.e. without fentanyl and diazepam. The results were then compared.

Table 3.Psychodiagnostic tests used to evaluate "street fitness" after anaesthesia

Sequence of tests	Test (apparatus)	Psychodiagnostic investigation	Time needed min.
1	Track-Tracer	Fine motor skilfulness, sensomotor coordination	2
2	Labyrinth (CHAPIUS)	Logical thinking and ability of co-ordination + combination	10
3	Counting test - count down 1000 to 975	Judgement + concentration	5
4	Reaction apparatus KIELER determination apparatus	Ability to react	2
5	Reaction apparatus (BECK) modified with physioscript (SCHWARZER)	Reaction speed	2
6	DÜKER (KLT)[+] counting test	Ability to concentrate and perform	30

[+] KLT = Konzentrations-Leistungs Test

Table 4. 10 Volunteers

Etomidate	0.30 mg/kg b.w. + Fentanyl 0.15 mg
Premedication	Atropin 0.5 mg + Diazepam 0.1 mg/kg b.w.
Etomidate	0.30 mg/kg b.w.
Premedication	Atropin 0.5 mg

Circulatory system, myocardial function, E.E.G.

Traffic-Fitness Test

Measuring of internal eye-pressure

Myocloni did not occur in the first group (Table 5). There was little change in sleep as compared to the reference group (KUGLER, DOENICKE, 1976). The ability to concentrate was not impaired two hours after anaesthesia with the test combination. Volunteers, however, turned out to be less discriminating, uninhibited and slightly euphoric. The same volunteers were efficient after etomidate without adjuncts and only showed some decrease in efficiency in

Table 5

	Myocloni	
Injection time	60 sec	60 sec
Premedication: Diazepam	0. 1 mg/kg b.w. i.v.	-
Doses: Etomidate + Fentanyl	0. 30 mg/kg b.w. 0. 15 mg	0.30 mg/kg b.w. -
n	10	10
Vp 1	O	+ + +
Vp 2	O	+ + +
Vp 3	O	+ + +
Vp 4	(+)	+ + +
Vp 5	O	+ + +
Vp 6	O	+ + +
Vp 7	O	O
Vp 8	O	+ + +
Vp 9	O	+ + +
Vp 10	O	+ + +

Myocloni: O = none
                  + = slight movements of the fingers only lasting for seconds
          + + + = heavy movements including other groups of muscles

track-tracing where fine-motor function and sensomotor coordination are tested. On the whole, however, they retained their critical ability and were not euphoric.

In view of these results patients can be discharged after two hours, if transport is provided. Permission to drive, however, should not be given for at least 12 hours because of the reduced capability of criticism. In investigations done afterwards, diazepam dosage was further reduced to 0.05 mg/kg b.w. (about 3. 5 mg). Even then myocloni did not occur. Although a post-narcotic tiredness was absent, patients should not be allowed to drive.

The pronounced myocloni in anaesthesias without any premedication confused us and other investigators in the beginning. The cause was soon found out by means of EEG examinations (DOENICKE et al., 1973) and various premedications (see also KUGLER and DOENICKE, 1976). Anaesthetists testing this new hypnotic for the first time clinically, should not let themselves be too much impressed with this symptom, because it becomes more and more insignificant in everyday routine.

The parallel tests of myocardial function showed no impairment with any of the combinations under investigation including reinjections. The fentanyl combination revealed a few cases of apnoea after the third injection, which, we think, was due to cumulation. Since a respirator with oxygen/nitrous oxide should always be available, respiration could be assisted in such cases.

As we found with our first studies on etomidate, a comparative test "clinical experiments with volunteers alternating with anaesthesia in patients" proved to be useful. Surgical interventions of short duration and diagnostical interventions in out-patients as well as minor operations of any type in in-patients were carried out after the following scheme of anaesthesia.

Premedication with diazepam 0.05 mg/kg b.w. - atropin 0.5 mg, etomidate 0.3 mg/kg b.w., + 0.15 mg fentanyl on average - both drugs being varied in dosage according to the general condition of the patient. Fentanyl may be mixed with etomidate in one syringe or better applied alone a little earlier. If the operation took more time, we either reinjected etomidate or made the patient inhale an oxygen/nitrous oxide mixture. If the hypnotic and analgesic effects were insufficient, etomidate and/or fentanyl could be reinjected at any time. Patients woke up soon and found anaesthesia pleasant. Out-patients could be discharged and taken home by car or ambulance 2 hours after the end of the operation.

The total number of etomidate anaesthesias for interventions of short duration (Table 6) carried out in our department (till 10.8.76) has been subdivided according to indication. Of particular interest seemed to be the repeated anaesthesias in patients receiving electro-shock. All 76 patients were pretreated with etomidate six times at short intervals. Allergic reactions occurred in none of the patients.

Table 6.Etomidate Short Narcosis

Surgery:	Incisions	339
	Reposition/Luxation	158
	Biopsies	100
	Removal of osteosynthesis material	6
Urology:	Cystoscopy	35
	Diathermia of papilloma	20
	Extraction of stones	9
Endoscopy:	Gastroscopy	78
	Rectoscopy	41
	Bronchoscopy	17
Angiography:		36
Cardioversion:		9
Gynaecological curettage:		834
Electro shock (76 patients x 6 anaesthesias)		456
Test persons		322
Total:		2460

A large number of out-patients underwent surgical interventions of short incisions and repositions. Many patients, one of them suffering from porphyria, had several etomidate anaesthesias. Complications such as allergic reactions and hypotension were not observed.

Summary

According to our experience in anaesthesias for interventions of short duration we intend to demonstrate possibilities for the use of etomidate. The fact that etomidate is not suitable as a mononarcotic is not considered as a drawback any longer because of its advantages as shown in thorough experimental work and extensive clinical experience. On the contrary, by using an individual dosage of hypnotic, analgesic and facultatively additional drugs we approached the primary ideal of a type of anaesthesia, which is as innocuous as possible and where each individual component is well controlled.

Zusammenfassung

Mit unseren Erfahrungen bei Narkosen für Kurzeingriffe sollten Möglichkeiten für den Einsatz von Etomidate aufgezeigt werden.

Daß es nicht als Mononarkotikum geeignet ist, erscheint uns bei den sonstigen, bisher gesicherten Vorteilen der Substanz nach gründlicher experimenteller Prüfung und jetzt bereits breiter klinischer Erfahrung kein Nachteil mehr zu sein. Im Gegenteil, durch die individuelle Dosierung von Hypnotikum, Analgetikum und evtl. anderer Adjuvantien sind wir dem alten Ideal einer möglichst unschädlichen, in allen Einzelfaktoren gut steuerbaren Anaesthesie wieder einen Schritt näher gekommen.

References

1. DOENICKE, A.: Street fitness after anaesthesia in out-patients. Acta anaesth. scand., Suppl. XVII, 95 (1965).

2. DOENICKE, A., KUGLER, J.: Prüfung eines neuen intravenösen Hypnoticums. Unveröffentlicht.

3. DOENICKE, A., KUGLER, J., PENZEL, G., LAUB, M., KILLIAN, I., KALMAR, L., BEZECNY, H.: Hirnfunktion und Toleranzbreite nach Etomidate, einem neuen barbituratfreien i.v. applizierbaren Hypnoticum. Anaesthesist 22, 357 (1973).

4. JANSSEN, P.A.J., NIEMEGEERS, C.J.E., SCHELLEKENS, K.H.L., LENAERTS, F.M.: Etomidate, R-(+)-Ethyl-1-($\propto$-methylbenzyl) imidazole-5-carboxylate (R 16659). Arzneimittel-Forsch. 21, 1234 (1971).

5. KUGLER, J., DOENICKE, A.: EEG after Etomidate. In: Anaesthesiologie und Wiederbelebung, Bd. 106. Berlin-Heidelberg-New York: Springer 1976.

Etomidate as "A New Drug in Intravenous Anaesthesia" (Conclusion)

A. Doenicke

Since March 1972, etomidate has been taken on clinical trial.
Metabolism occurs quickly. Up to now, there was no evidence of
histamine release or immunodepressant effect either in biochemical investigations or in clinical tests. A final conclusion,
however, should only be made after many years of clinical experience. As shown in the EEG, the deep stages of narcosis are similar
to those of barbiturates. The absence of analgesia and frequency
of myocloni during etomidate narcosis make us assume that, unlike
with barbiturates, there is no inhibition of the thalamic (diencephalic) region or of any subthalamic structures.
Using etomidate, KUGLER and DOENICKE induced general anaesthesia
for surgical treatment in 4 patients with cerebral convulsions.
Then, no motoric or epileptic signs could be seen. The simultaneously registered EEG did not show any paroxysmal electroencephalographic activities. No activation of a characteristic discharge
pattern could be detected pointing to a possible epileptogenic
potency of etomidate.
Similar deliberations were made concerning ketanest and certain
halogenated hydrocarbon compounds. A direct pharmacodynamic
epileptogenic effect has not yet been proved.
Comparing dosages being commonly used in clinical practice, the
hypnotic effect of etomidate (0.3 mg/kg b.w.) is stronger than
that of methohexital (1.5 mg/kg b.w.), thiopental (5 mg/kg b.w.)
or propanidid (5 mg/kg b.w.).

The best way to abolish side-effects like involuntary muscle
movements, myocloni, is to use substances, which mainly influence
those structures being less affected by etomidate. Small doses
of fentanyl suppress the interfering myocloni considered as a
sign of non-restrained subcortical structures. Therefore, premedication with a psychotropic drug (diazepam 0.5 mg/kg b.w.) and
fentanyl (0.05 - 0.1 mg), an analgesic, is indicated.

In addition, venous pain and involuntary muscle movements were
seen as main-effects of etomidate in a multinational study. They
are not necessarily harmful but inconvenient. It should be noted
that until now all studies were performed with etomidate as a
sulfate salt reconstituted to an isotonic and buffered solution.

A recently completed pilot study promised that pain of injection
and muscle movements will be greatly reduced or totally overcome
if a solution of etomidate base in 35 % propylene glycol is used.
Besides, the extent of side-effects directly correlates with the
intensity of venous pain (see appendix).

Haemodynamics are little affected by etomidate. After injection
of O.3 mg/kg b.w. etomidate, there is a rise in cardiac output,
cardiac index, heart rate. Mean arterial pressure, peripheral
vascular resistance and dp/dt max. decrease slightly. After a
few minutes, all parameters return to normal. Despite the small
influence on blood gases, assisting respiration should be available.

During the past few years the effect of anaesthetics on liver
function was more and more emphasized. Therefore, it is important
to know how a substance effects liver function even after having
repeatedly been administered. In this context the results of GÖTZ
(1974) are worth mentioning. He investigates oxygen consumption
and gluconeogenesis by perfusing isolated rat livers. Unlike
with barbiturates, Halothane and Ethrane, no changes have been
found in these parameters at etomidate concentrations within
the range of clinical use. Only at very high concentrations a
decrease in oxygen consumption was measured. However, this was
quickly and completely reversible.

According to our own experience, liver function remains unaffected
even after repeated anaesthesia (7 times within a few weeks).

In JANSSEN's opinion, an induction of microsomal liver enzymes
cannot be detected. As numerous anaesthetists miss a hypnotic
component in NLA a combination with either diazepam, ketamine,
propanidid, barbiturates or RO 5O 422 (a derivate of diazepam)
has been recommended. Because of its pharmacological profile, its
absence or limited effect on the cardiovascular system and its
wide range of hypnotic tolerance, etomidate is predestined for
induction of NLA. Consumption of DHB would be economized. Also
for induction of Halothane and Ethrane anaesthesias, etomidate
offers more advantages in comparison to the former intravenous
anaesthetics.

Experiences in open heart surgery showed better results when using
etomidate for induction of narcosis. There will be only slight
influence on an insufficient heart. In such cases a lower dosage
is indicated, because of a transient drop in blood pressure
due to a decrease of peripheral vascular resistance and mean
arterial pressure.

Even in one of our first narcoses in 1972 when treating a patient
nearly bled to death who had suffered from a short cardiac arrest,
we already realized a wide range of tolerance of that drug. During
a subsequent emergency operation (extensive treatment) narcosis
was maintained by reinjection of etomidate and fentanyl as an
analgesic for more than 1 1/2 hours.

PETER (Mannheim/München) did comparative studies on several drugs
using a shock model. He found etomidate having the least side
effects on shocked patients.

Problems of short narcosis are as follows:
Being a pure hypnotic, etomidate is not suitable for mono-narcosis.
The usefulness of an anaesthetic for out-patients depends on its

possible impairment of efficiency and concentration power after
narcosis. 90 minutes after injecting a combination of diazepam
0.05 mg/kg b.w., fentanyl 0.15 mg and etomidate 0.3 mg/kg b.w.,
the capability to concentrate was only slightly affected.

Since propanidid and barbiturates are both not free from side-
effects and do not possess an analgesic component, a combination
of etomidate/fentanyl for out-patients anaesthesia has more
advantages in comparison to former methods commonly being in
clinical use.

By using individual doses of hypnotic, analgesic and perhaps
additional drugs (N_2O/O_2) we have approached the ideal of anaesthesia being as innocuous as possible and easily controlled in
all its components.

Appendix

A multinational study shows the dependence of pain during injection on premedication as well as on dosages and speed of injection.

This investigation is based on the analysis of 4763 case reports
of 45 anaesthetists from 9 countries (V. SCHUERMANS et al). 12.9 %
of 4452 patients complained of venous pain, the least after premedication with fentanyl or innovar, i.e. Thalamonal. This correlates well with our own results.

Whereas in our study a constant dose of 0.2 mg etomidate/kg b.w.
was given, the frequency of venous pain in relation to the dosage
was analysed in the multinational study. Incidence of venous pain
is parallel to increase of dosage (from 9.2 % to approx. 21.8 %
at double dosage).

It is understandable that the stimulus of pain significantly
increases tachycardia from 3.7 to 9.4 %.

Furthermore, the percental increase of muscle movements, especially of myocloni, is of clinical interest.

Their aggravation is highly significant if the patients felt pain
during injection. In detail:

Among the patients who had no injection pain, 9.4 % showed slight
and 4.2 % strong myocloni. Among those who complained of venous
pain slight myocloni were observed in 22.3 % and strong ones in
10.1 %.

Thus, the multinational study shows that:

- the administration of i.v. fentanyl in the induction phase
  just before etomidate significantly reduces the incidence of
  all involuntary muscle movements

- The venous pain of injection is dependent on the diameter of the vein (in our study: 1 % in the V. basilica and 11 - 12 % on the dorsum of the hand) and not associated with thrombophlebitis.

- Involuntary muscle movements are a consequence of both the venous pain of injection and the lack of analgesic properties.

Anaesthesiology and Resuscitation · Anaesthesiologie und Wiederbelebung
Anesthésiologie et Réanimation

Editors: R. Frey, F. Kern, O. Mayrhofer. Managing Editor: H. Bergmann

Eine Auswahl lieferbarer Bände:

1 Resuscitation. Controversial Aspects. Edited by Peter Safar. VII, 64 pages. DM 26,–. 1963

2 Hypnosis in Anaesthesiology. Edited by Jean Lassner. VIII, 51 Seiten. DM 24,–. 1964

5 Infusionsprobleme in der Chirurgie. Herausgegeben von U. F. Gruber. VIII, 108 Seiten. DM 14,–. 1968

6 Parenterale Ernährung. Herausgegeben von K. Lang, R. Frey und M. Halmágyi. X, 156 Seiten. DM 34,–. 1966

7 Grundlagen und Ergebnisse der Venendruckmessung zur Prüfung des zirkulierenden Blutvolumens. Von V. Feurstein. VIII, 37 Seiten. DM 19,–. 1965

11 Der Elektrolytstoffwechsel von Hirngewebe und seine Beeinflussung durch Narkotica. Von W. Klaus. VIII, 97 Seiten. DM 33,–. 1967

12 Sauerstoffversorgung und Säure-Basenhaushalt in tiefer Hypothermie. Von P. Lundsgaard-Hansen. VIII, 91 Seiten. DM 30,–. 1966

14 Die Technik der Lokalanaesthesie. Von H. Nolte. VIII, 53 Seiten. DM 14,–. 1966

15 Anaesthesie und Notfallmedizin. Herausgegeben von K. Hutschenreuter. XII, 286 Seiten. DM 78,–. 1966

16 Anaesthesiologische Probleme in der HNO-Heilkunde und Kieferchirurgie. Herausgegeben von K. Horatz und H. Kreuscher. VIII, 39 Seiten. DM 19,–. 1966

19 Örtliche Betäubung: Plexus brachialis. Von Sir Robert R. Macintosh und W. W. Mushin. VIII, 32 Seiten. DM 20,–. 1967

20 Anaesthesie in der Gefäß- und Herzchirurgie. Herausgegeben von O. H. Just und M. Zindler. XII, 209 Seiten. DM 64,–. 1967

21 Die Hirndurchblutung unter Neuroleptanaesthesie. Von H. Kreuscher. VIII, 85 Seiten. DM 33,–. 1967

22 Ateminsuffizienz. Von H. L'Allemand. VIII, 90 Seiten. DM 36,–. 1968

23 Die Geschichte der chirurgischen Anaesthesie. Von Thomas E. Keys. XVIII, 230 Seiten. DM 78,–. 1968

24 Ventilation und Atemtechnik bei Säuglingen und Kleinkindern unter Narkosebedingungen. Von J. Wawersik. X, 151 Seiten. DM 52,–. 1967

25 Morphinartige Analgetika und ihre Antagonisten. Von Francis F. Foldes, Mark Swerdlow, and Ephraim S. Siker. XXIII, 364 Seiten. DM 110,–. 1968

26 Örtliche Betäubung: Kopf und Hals. Von Sir Robert R. Macintosh und M. Ostler. VIII, 124 Seiten. DM 67,–. 1968

27 Langzeitbeatmung. Herausgegeben von Ch. Lehmann. XIV, 91 Seiten. DM 39,–. 1968

28 Die Wiederbelebung der Atmung. Von H. Nolte. XII, 89 Seiten. DM 14,–. 1968

29 Kontrolle der Ventilation in der Neugeborenen- und Säuglingsanaesthesie. Von U. Henneberg. VII, 73 Seiten. DM 34,–. 1968

30 Hypoxie. Herausgegeben von R. Frey, M. Halmágyi, Karl Lang und G. Thews. X, 176 Seiten. DM 69,–. 1969

32 Örtliche Betäubung: Abdominal-Chirurgie. Von Sir Robert R. Macintosh und R. Bryce-Smith. XI, 73 Seiten. DM 62,–. 1968

33 Planung, Organisation und Einrichtung von Intensivbehandlungseinheiten am Krankenhaus. Herausgegeben von H. W. Opderbecke. X, 230 Seiten. DM 49,–. 1969

35 Die Störungen des Säure-Basen-Haushaltes. Herausgegeben von V. Feurstein. X, 149 Seiten. DM 56,–. 1969

36 Anaesthesie und Nierenfunktion. Herausgegeben von V. Feurstein. X, 142 Seiten. DM 53,–. 1969

37 Anaesthesie und Kohlenhydratstoffwechsel. Herausgegeben von V. Feurstein. VIII, 83 Seiten. DM 36,–. 1969

38 Respiratorbeatmung und Oberflächenspannung in der Lunge. Von H. Benzer. IX, 51 Seiten. DM 24,–. 1969

39 Die nasotracheale Intubation. Von M. Körner. XI, 94 Seiten. DM 43,–. 1969

41 Über das Verhalten von Ventilation, Gasaustausch und Kreislauf bei Patienten mit normalem und gestörtem Gasaustausch unter künstlicher Totraumvergrößerung. Von O. Giebel. VII, 74 Seiten. DM 26,–. 1969

43 Die Klinik des Wundstarrkrampfes im Lichte neuzeitlicher Behandlungsmethoden. Von K. Eyrich. VIII, 95 Seiten. DM 30,–. 1969

45 Vergiftungen. Erkennung, Verhütung und Behandlung. Herausgegeben von R. Frey, M. Halmágyi, K. Lang und P. Oettel. XX, 173 Seiten. DM 30,–. 1970

46 Veränderungen des Wasser- und Elektrolythaushaltes durch Osmotherapeutika. Von M. Halmágyi. XII, 77 Seiten. DM 30,–. 1970

48 Intensivtherapie bei Kreislaufversagen. Herausgegeben von S. Effert und K. Wiemers. IX, 108 Seiten. DM 43,–. 1970

50 Intensivtherapie beim septischen Schock. Herausgegeben von F. W. Ahnefeld und M. Halmágyi. IX, 103 Seiten. DM 44,–. 1970

51 Prämedikationseffekte auf Bronchialwiderstand und Atmung. Von L. Stöcker. VII, 46 Seiten. DM 26,–. 1971

52 Die Bedeutung der adrenergen Blockade für den haemorrhagischen Schock. Von G. Zierott. VIII, 115 Seiten. DM 62,–. 1971

53 Nomogramme zum Säure-Basen-Status des Blutes und zum Atemgastransport. Herausgegeben von G. Thews, XI, 134 Seiten. DM 48,–. 1971

56 Anaesthesie bei Eingriffen an endokrinen Organen und bei Herzrhythmusstörungen. Herausgegeben von K. Hutschenreuter und M. Zindler. XII, 223 Seiten. DM 47,–. 1972

58 Stoffwechsel. Pathophysiologische Grundlagen der Intensivtherapie. Herausgegeben von K. Lang, R. Frey und M. Halmágyi. X, 142 Seiten. DM 59,–. 1972

59 Anaesthesia Equipment. By P. Schreiber. XII, 219 pages. DM 59,–. 1972

60 Homoiostase. Wiederherstellung und Aufrechterhaltung. Herausgegeben von F. W. Ahnefeld und M. Halmágyi. XI, 192 Seiten. DM 83,–. 1972

61 Essays on Future Trends in Anaesthesia. By A. Boba. X, 93 pages. DM 36,–. 1972

62 Respiratorischer Flüssigkeits- und Wärmeverlust des Säuglings und Kleinkindes bei künstlicher Beatmung. Von W. Dick. VIII, 69 Seiten. DM 40,–. 1972

64 Sauerstoffüberdruckbehandlung. Probleme und Anwendung. Herausgegeben von I. Podlesch. IX, 97 Seiten. DM 47,–. 1972

65 Der Wasser- und Elektrolythaushalt des Kranken. Von H. Baur. XI, 221 Seiten. DM 59,–. 1972

66 Überlebens- und Wiederbelebungszeit des Herzens. Von P. G. Spieckermann. IX, 116 Seiten. DM 47,–. 1973

67 Sauerstoffbedarf und Sauerstoffversorgung des Herzens in Narkose. Von D. Kettler. VIII, 53 Seiten. DM 30,–. 1973

68 Anaesthesie mit Gamma-Hydroxibuttersäure. Herausgegeben von W. Bushart und P. Rittmeyer. IX, 93 Seiten. DM 30,–. 1973

70 Die Sekretionsleistung des Nebennierenmarks unter dem Einfluß von Narkotica und Muskelrelaxantien. Von M. Göthert. VIII, 89 Seiten. DM 36,–. 1972

71 Anaesthesie und Wiederbelebung bei Säuglingen und Kleinkindern. Herausgegeben von F. W. Ahnefeld und M. Halmágyi. IX, 83 Seiten. DM 40,–. 1973

72 Therapie lebensbedrohlicher Zustände bei Säuglingen und Kleinkindern. Herausgegeben von R. Frey, M. Halmágyi und K. Lang. IX, 136 Seiten. DM 69,–. 1973

73 Diagnostische und therapeutische Nervenblockaden. Herausgegeben von R. Frey, M. Halmágyi und H. Nolte. IX, 67 Seiten. DM 36,–. 1973

75 Anesthetic Management of Endocrine Disease. By T. Oyama. IX, 220 pages. DM 65,–. 1973

77 Herzrhythmus und Anaesthesie. Herausgegeben von H. Nolte und J. Wurster. IX, 55 Seiten. DM 30,–. 1973

78 Biotelemetrie. Angewandte biomedizinische Technik. Von H. Hutten. VII, 70 Seiten. DM 39,–. 1973

79 Coronardurchblutung und Energieumsatz des menschlichen Herzens unter verschiedenen Anaesthetica. Von H. Sonntag. VIII, 56 Seiten. DM 36,–. 1973

80 Anaesthesie. Atmung – Kreislauf. Herausgegeben von M. Gemperle, G. Hossli und B. Tschirren. XIII, 278 Seiten. DM 58,–. 1974

81 Stoffwechselwirkungen von Trometamol. Von H. Helwig. VIII, 96 Seiten. DM 36,–. 1974

82 Engström-Respirator. Herausgegeben von G. Kalff und P. Herzog. X, 105 Seiten. DM 38,–. 1974

84 Ethrane. Edited by P. Lawin und R. Beer in cooperation with E. Wiethoff. XIII, 389 pages. DM 64,–. 1974

85 Blutersatz durch stromafreie Hämoglobinlösung. Von J. M. Unseld. VIII, 90 Seiten. DM 32,–. 1974

95 Mobile Intensive Care Units. Edited by R. Frey, E. Nagel and P. Safar. XV, 271 pages. DM 48,–. 1976

98 Intraaortale Ballongegenpulsation. Von E. R. de Vivie. X, 96 Seiten. DM 28,–. 1976

99 Inhalationsanaesthesie mit Ethrane. Herausgegeben von J. B. Brückner. XII, 254 Seiten. DM 48,–. 1976

101 Myokarddurchblutung und Stoffwechselparameter im arteriellen Blut bei Hämodilutionsperfusion. Von D. Regensburger. VII, 75 Seiten. DM 36,–. 1976

102 Coronarinsuffizienz, Pathophysiologie und Anaesthesieprobleme bei der Coronarchirurgie. Herausgegeben von M. Zindler und R. Purschke. XIII, 166 Seiten. DM 48,–. 1977

103 Fettemulsionen in der parenteralen Ernährung. Herausgegeben von A. Wretlind, R. Frey, K. Eyrich und H. Makowski. X, 222 Seiten. DM 48,–. 1977

104 Die akute normovolämische Hämodilution in klinischer Anwendung. Von A. J. Coburg. XI, 89 Seiten. DM 28,–. 1977

105 Lungenveränderungen während Dauerbeatmung. Von H. Reineke. VII, 56 Seiten. DM 36,–. 1977

107 Die kontrollierte Hypotension mit Nitroprussidnatrium in der Neuroanaesthesie. Von K. Huse. IX, 98 Seiten. DM 38,–. 1977

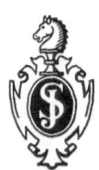

Preisänderungen vorbehalten

Springer-Verlag Berlin   Heidelberg   New York